Flies in My Coffee

M. Rene Harris

Published by Richter Publishing LLC www.richterpublishing.com

Book Cover Photos: Pierce Brunson Photography

Editors: MD Weems, Diana Fisler, Kay Karolyshyn, & Elaine Ralford

ISBN: 1945812028

ISBN-13:9781945812026

DISCLAIMER

This book is designed to provide information on relationships only. This information is provided and sold with the knowledge that the publisher and author do not offer any legal or medical advice. In the case of a need for any such expertise consult with the appropriate professional. This book does not contain all information available on any subject. This book has not been created to be specific to any individual people or organization's situation or needs. Reasonable efforts have been made to make this book as accurate as possible. However, there may be typographical and or content errors. Therefore, this book should serve only as general entertainment. This book contains information that might be dated or erroneous and is intended only to educate and entertain. The author and publisher shall have no liability or responsibility to any person or entity regarding any loss or damage incurred, or alleged to have incurred, directly or indirectly, by the information contained in this book or as a result of anyone acting or failing to act upon the information in this book. You hereby agree never to sue and to hold the author and publisher harmless from any and all claims arising out of the information contained in this book. You hereby agree to be bound by this disclaimer, covenant not to sue and release. You may return this book within the guarantee time period for a full refund. In the interest of full disclosure, this book contains affiliate links that might pay the author or publisher a commission upon any purchase from the company. While the author and publisher take no responsibility for any virus or technical issues that could be caused by such links, the business practices of these companies and or the performance of any product or service, the author or publisher has used the product or service and makes a recommendation in good faith based on that experience. All characters appearing in this work are fictitious. Any resemblance to real persons, living or dead, is purely coincidental. The opinions and stories in this book are the views of the author and not that of the publisher.

M. Rene Harris

DEDICATION

Thank you to my beautiful children, for believing in my stories and giving me the very best job in the whole world! I couldn't do this without you—and I wouldn't want to. Thank you for being a part of my journey. You are more valuable than you know.

M. Rene Harris

CONTENTS

M. Rene Harris

ACKNOWLEDGMENTS

Thank you to Dr. Karen Dyer who saved my son's life. I am forever grateful to have you as a friend.

M. Rene Harris

INTRODUCTION

Sometimes we find ourselves in situations that we would never dream we'd find ourselves in. After all, we're intelligent, loving and caring people. Right? Too smart to find ourselves on the other end of the abusive carrot and stick, the intermittent reinforcement syndrome. Yet here I was, in an experience most would easily judge or gossip about.

It's the inevitable hindsight of "WTF was I thinking" after the relationship is over that can be even more devastating. It defies reason and logic to stay in a situation where your mind cannot find recourse of action or a defense of your self-esteem. Only now as I write this book, have I learned what an expert I had become at playing the martyr. This role became almost my internal badge of honor, a silent martyr. I learned only too well to sacrifice myself. I gave up my voice, my feelings, and my happiness.

I learned that I can only give my children that which I have myself and I was empty with such a deep void, so deep that I could no longer see past what had become familiar. Its familiarity had become my comfort zone in a distorted way merely because of recognition. How much damage had I done to my children knowing that our adult relationships and how we interact with them are formed as early as age three and that the first five years, the formative years, are critical in shaping a child's personality and psyche and emotional well-being. Since how parents relate to one another and more importantly how they relate to us, teaches us to relate to others, what was my staying in an abusive relationship teaching my children? Do I teach them that I took my vows seriously, "for better or for worse"?

Do I teach them that commitment means doing the things you said you would do long after the mood disappears? Or do I teach them that even God expects you to have some semblance of happiness and that my model of abuse which they experience daily in our home is not one I want them to perpetuate. This constant internal conflict tugged at me and kept me immobilized.

I came to recognize that my suffering was an inside job, that no one was responsible for the condition and position that I was allowing to paralyze me but myself. I had to take full responsibility for my own life. In my search for myself, I turned to my God. But the God in whom I grew up believing was limiting and punishing and worst of all judging. I needed no more judgment as no one judged me more harshly than I judged myself. This word God was contaminated by so much social and religious conditioning that I could no longer relate to It.

I read, meditated, begged, and pleaded for some relief, some external Source, to drive my energy in the right direction. When I couldn't find a word higher than that which I referred to as God, I finally found the energy of the Empyreal Pull. Somehow in its abstraction, and unfamiliarity, this phrase had tangible and concrete meaning for me. Empyreal Pull is an energy of pure fire and light. An energy so refined beyond a real substance that it pertains to the highest and purest region of Heaven. In this Empyreal Pull, I found my voice, my power, myself! It is this Light that showed me a healthier path.

It is only through this Light that I found my vision. It is this Light that gave me back my eyes, my senses and allowed me to invest in myself. This light cast on the shadows of myself allowing me to see how very emotionally bankrupt I had become. Allowing me to build my emotional bank account so I could release myself from the prison in which I placed myself. It is in this Light that I learned to be still and silent. Only in this stillness did I find myself. Only in this stillness and in this silence, did I recognize my shadows. Only in my shadows could I begin to heal myself. Learning these lessons took years of waking up but not before it almost took my sanity.

Ultimately, it is about empowerment. It's about knowing where it is that you can take action to create positive changes in your life and know where it is we must surrender. Understanding where your power is and how to recognize it is what propels us beyond our current state of inertia. In the shadows, we go from victim to rescuer, and then to martyr. A vicious cycle that never seems to end in the name of sacrificing ourselves for the greater good of everyone else but ourselves, a role I had assumed long before my marriage. I brought this pattern into all my relationships, into my marriage, my job, and all my interpersonal relationships. Then after feeling all used up, one day I awakened!

The flies in my coffee were the catalyst that took me from the nightmare in which I had placed myself and Pulled me into my awakening. Today I cannot see a fly without offering gratitude for the part they played in my transformation. The flies in your coffee offer a sign to help guide you to a more developed understanding of how your life could be. It is Spirit working to move you towards greater love. Love for yourself and those around you. Towards forgiveness of those who you could not imagine meeting with ultimate forgiveness.

Through my story, my desire, and intention is for people to understand the powerful dynamic of intermittent reinforcement that can keep us stuck in situations that do not serve our highest potential. I pray that my book will help you seek and find your Pull and your strength to take the steps to become victorious in your own life. If my story helps even one soul on his or her journey, then this book has been a pure success. May you all be blessed and see only abundance in your lives

"We ask ourselves, 'Who am I to be brilliant, gorgeous, talented, fabulous?' Actually, who are you not to be? You are a child of God. Your playing small does not serve the world. There is nothing enlightened about shrinking so that other people won't feel insecure around you." ~ *Marianne Williamson*

CHAPTER ONE

Blurred Lines

"Innocence ends when one is stripped of the delusion that one likes oneself." ~ Joan Didion

I woke up and with my eyes still closed, I took a deep breath. Without opening my eyes, I lay there for a moment. Still. Not moving. Breathing. It seemed like any ordinary day, but this day would prove to be anything but. I opened my eyes and saw him, just lying there. Sleeping, snoring. I scrunched my face in disgust. I hated him. I never wanted to feel this way, but I now feel a disdain for this stranger lying next to me. I wondered what kind of mood he would be in today. We never knew what to expect or the temperament that would dictate our day. *I will leave him, just not yet,* I promised myself as I lay there. *But first, I'd have to strategize a plan. A solid, fool proof plan to survive.*

What would happen today would become just the latest blow in a long line of damaging strikes to my self-esteem. But this is not where my story begins. Not by a long shot.

I was 18, and had trouble finding a job that paid enough to please my parents, but that day I had an interview as a dancer in a nightclub downtown. I can't believe I'm doing this, but I need a job. Even though I live in my parents' house, they made it very clear that I need to earn my keep. My father had given me the receipt for the Kotex he bought me expecting to be fully reimbursed. I had just started Community College to study Interior Design. I was studying at night and selling portrait packages by Olan Mills during the day. I was doing pretty good but soon discovered that I was not making enough to pay for classes at the college and afford the simple things a girl needs, like Kotex. My girlfriend told me this place was hiring. She had just started working there and wanted to recruit me.

"You can make a lot of money dancing, and you wouldn't have to do it forever."

"What kind of dancing? Do I have to get naked?"

"No, just show your boobs."

"I don't have big boobs, but I do like dancing, so it can't be that bad."

I had taken a dance class in high school, but I was pretty sure that was not the kind of dancing Krista was referring to. I recalled the only type of exotic dancing I had ever seen. Burlesque! I had seen it on TV. The kind of dancing that was a slow strip tease and the ultimate "ta-da" was the revealing of the boobs and those usually had tassels covering the nipples. I stood in the mirror wondering how in the hell you make tassels twirl around.

It was late morning the next day when Krista was to meet me at the club.

As I was getting dressed, I danced around the house practicing my best moves. Then I stopped. I stood still in my grandmother's living room and became fixed on the backyard which sprawled out for a little less than a quarter of an acre. From the sliding glass door just off the patio, I noticed a man in the yard, he was spraying something on the grass. He was average height, blond hair and shirtless. I heard a voice in my ear say, "That's your husband." I laughed to myself thinking "I wish," and I danced off to finish getting dressed and apply my makeup the best I could for an 18-year-old. I was off to get a job as an exotic dancer. It felt like an adventure. I felt a nervous excitement rise up within me, however, my naiveté had in no way prepared me for what was about to take place in my life.

It didn't take long for me to realize that I hated doing this. This wasn't me – it wasn't right. It wasn't what I wanted to be doing. My audience grew, and at first, I must admit that I did enjoy the creepy attention. I certainly enjoyed the money and I did make a lot. Some nights I went home with over $500 in cash. That was an enormous amount of money to me at my age. It was mine and I was able to hand my parents cash when they asked for it and they asked no questions about where I had gotten the money.

I had never really had a real drink except for the few times I would sneak some of my parents' liquor when they weren't home. I never cared for the taste of it. One night Krista asked me to try what she was drinking. It was sweet with a little kick. "It's called a Long Island Iced Tea."

"Does it have any tea in it?"

"I don't know," she said shrugging her shoulders. So I ordered my own. After drinking only half of it I felt a little bolder. A little less judged by all the horny faces gawking at me. Doing this felt wrong for me, but it also made me feel desirable in a sleazy sort of way. I began to use my newly discovered liquid courage just so that I could dance. The novelty of all of it had worn off quickly and I found that I could not do this without first numbing my moral senses, with that Long Island Iced Tea. One night I was dancing and as I looked out into the club, I saw someone that made my heart stop.

My brother!

Of all the people in the world, my brother was sitting out there looking at me - looking at him. My brother saw me! Now he was threatening to tell my parents if I didn't let him use my car at his will. That night, my blackmailer took control of my car and left.

At the end of the night, I had one Long Island Iced tea while waiting for his return, but this time, I felt weird. I felt drunk, very drunk, very quickly and I didn't even finish the drink. I figured maybe it was because I had not eaten and the liquor had gone straight to my head. The owner of the club, Mr. Nelson, offered to take me home and I thought that was really nice of him. On the way home, he stated he had to stop and meet Joe, the club's promoter. He needed to pick up something from him. I knew Joe, he was a nice guy and was very protective of me when I was at the club. He prevented men from touching me or pulling me off the stage. He would have men removed from the club at the wave of my hand. I was often reminded to use that power sparingly because they were paying customers after all.

I wasn't feeling well when we arrived at the "meeting place" where Joe was to be; it was a motel in a location that I was not familiar with. I looked at Mr. Nelson and told him I wanted to go home. I told him I felt sick. He told me not to worry, that we would only be a few minutes, that Joe was inside and he was just going in to grab something and then he would take me home. He promised. I still felt uneasy inside and tried to will myself to become sober. To think. To get control. NOW!

"Come on in and say hi to Joe." He motioned with his hand for me to follow him as he got out of the car. I hesitantly followed

Mr. Nelson to the door of the room. I told myself to remember the room number. Remember the name of the hotel. When Mr. Nelson knocked on the door and Joe opened it, I felt immediately relaxed and all but forgot the fight or flight sensation that my body had warned me about only moments ago.

He was friendly and smiled and invited us in. I looked around the room and saw Sheryl, another dancer from the club, sitting on one of the two beds that were positioned in the middle of the room. I greeted her and covered the fact that my gut was telling me something was not right.

Mr. Nelson and Joe went over to the desk in the large room and went through some papers. I moved over to the bed where Sheryl was sitting and tried to strike up a friendly conversation when I noticed that her words were slurring and her eyes were glassy. I turned to look at the men who brought us to this room and Joe seemed to have miraculously appeared at the bed where Sheryl and I were sitting.

He laid Sheryl back and began kissing her, she did not fight him. She was a willing participant. I got up quickly as I thought we must certainly be leaving now to let Joe and Sheryl continue their thing, whatever that was. As I began to walk briskly towards the door, Mr. Nelson grabbed me by the hand and tried to pull me towards him as he stepped back and sat on the bed. He now had both of my hands and was pulling me towards him. As he sat on the bed, I screamed, "I WANT TO GO HOME! I WANT TO GO HOME!"

Joe and Sheryl shot up and Sheryl said, "Just take her home." With that, Mr. Nelson grabbed his keys and we left. The ride seemed to take forever and not a word was spoken. When we arrived at my parents' home, Mr. Nelson pulled into the driveway and stopped but kept the car running. He looked at me and told me he was very sorry. I simply looked at him, exited the car, walked into the house and threw up all over the kitchen floor.

I went back to the club a few nights later to get my things and my final pay; my friend Krista went with me. As I waited for Mr. Nelson to arrive, Krista and I sat at the bar and next to us sat a man with blond hair and the most piercing blue eyes I'd ever seen. Krista struck up a conversation with him and they seemed to hit it off. As we were getting ready to leave, I discovered my car was gone. My brother had taken it again. Damn it! How did he even know I was there?

The man with the ice blue eyes overheard our conversation and offered to give us a ride. While I was hesitant, Krista happily accepted for the both of us. He introduced himself as Albert and said he was leaving anyway and offered to get us something to eat on the way because he was hungry. We made a quick stop at the Taco Bell drive-thru, and then headed off to my house to drop me off first so that they could continue their discussion together alone. In the front seat, I gave directions and he drove speaking to Krista in the back seat. As we neared my neighborhood, he commented that he worked over here sometimes.

As we pulled up to my parent's house, he stated that he had been to this house before. He knew this house. I asked him how he knew. He told me that he worked in pest control and he was at this house about a month ago spraying the back yard for fleas. I told him that he should probably wear a shirt next time he does that. He laughed and I left. It would be another two weeks before he came to my parents' house again, but this time, he would be looking for me.

Flies in My Coffee

CHAPTER TWO

Know Thyself

"What a gloomy thing, not to know the address of one's soul."
~ Victor Hugo.

Albert wasn't the tall, dark and handsome type. He was rugged and charismatic with piercing blue eyes and a hypnotic smile. Something about him had me hooked. He was different. Uncultured, reckless and a little rude. He was everything different than I was, everything different than I had ever known. We started seeing each other regularly and after a few months of what I thought was dating, I began to believe that maybe he wasn't as serious about me as I was about him. My parents did not approve when they finally met him. I thought it was because Albert was white and we were black even though my parents had never shown any racist signs. We lived overseas as I was growing up and I was raised to embrace all types of different cultures and ethnicities. We had always been taught to be tolerant of people's differences even if they didn't accept ours. But when it came to Albert, there was a very clear difference in my parent's behavior. I felt that they just didn't understand him. If they could only get to know him, I was sure they would change their minds. Albert and I would plan dates and I was often stood up because he "forgot." If we did go out somewhere, it was to house parties or pool parties with his friends who were equally rude, uncultured and reckless. I didn't see it at the time. He was allowed to have his own life after all or was I being "Friend Zoned?" I didn't know, but he was present and charming and so darned cute.

Since I had quit my dancing job, I needed another job and I decided to go into the military. I needed a change. I also needed to get away from this bad boy who had been consuming my thoughts and my time for nearly a year.

I enlisted in the Marine Corps that summer and Albert would write regularly while I was in boot camp. I began looking forward to mail call on Sunday morning, always hoping there would be something there for me. When there was, I was elated. I would run to my bunk and lay there and read Albert's words of encouragement over and over. Every now and then, I would get a letter from my dad, telling me how proud he was of me and to hang in there. But nothing grips your heart and soul like words of love from a man who you believe to be waiting for you.

When your mind is being reshaped and remolded, when you are being broken and rebuilt, whatever influence there is in your life at that time becomes part of your new being. The severity in which the spirit is broken by the U.S. Marine Corps is the same severity in which you are rebuilt. I was programmed to be blindly loyal to those in authority over me no matter the mission. I was being programmed to fight for that undying loyalty at all costs. That is what keeps us alive. You do or you die. I didn't learn to depend on a man, I learned to be loyal to one. Forever faithful.

I had developed a backbone. A sense of pride that I had never known before. My physical body had been pushed to limits I didn't know was possible. It would be many years later that I would discover the mental and physical transformation that was happening to me now, would solidify itself into becoming my new being. I was a new person, stronger in many ways and so much weaker in others.

Breaking the human spirit is one thing. Rebuilding that spirit is something else. I was rebuilt with things like pride and judgment, camaraderie and dedication, loyalty and a sense of justice. I watched many women broken into little girls and was determined not to be one of them. Some broke quickly, some over time.

Basic training was not really about training people at all. It's about changing everything you've already been taught to believe. It's changing you so that you believe that you can do things you wouldn't have dreamed you were capable of doing.

Training a young woman to perform under the threat of death and extreme pressure and defies all logic, it goes against our very instinct and takes the most intensive acts of psychological reprogramming to overcome. You may never overcome the intense draw towards danger. It is now a part of you.

The threat and the feeling of assault was there even though the drill instructors never physically touched you. Standing nose to nose while they verbally degraded your existence served to test your resolve. You soon appreciate that it's not about making you feel stupid or small or incapable, it is about something else entirely different. But it still makes you want to fight back resulting in a building up a desire to fight back. To protect and defend yourself but you stuff that down. You hold it in until you are allowed to unleash the fight. And when the time comes, may God help the ones who that box is unleashed on. It's about becoming deprogrammed and reprogrammed both psychologically and physically to make you a Marine.

What a brilliant form of psychological training. The ability to break and rebuild anyone who thinks they can't be broken. It placed within me a sense that I was expected to do something far more important than anything expected from other ordinary people.

Imagine all of this happening during one of the most intensely stressful periods of anybody's life, young adulthood. That transition from childhood and dependence to adulthood and independence. I was taught that everything I was before now was weak and absent of any real value. Cults possess this same type of programmed mindset. This psychological transformation is as intense and intentional as any cult or religion. From this point on, I will be different and have this indescribable culture as part of my new psyche, forever.

The erosion of my individuality starts by separating you from everything that makes you who you are. My tribe, my family, my friends, environment, beliefs, and all of its rituals and traditions are no longer recognizable as the norm. I lost my entire individuality, everything that I thought made me special and unique. That entity that I came to believe that made me valuable. My role in this world had changed.

Whatever it was that, as a young adult gave me the innate desire to stretch my wings and be a grown up, the thing that made me feel that I was better than the orders I might have received from my parents or anyone else in authority over me, was being stripped away. Whatever it was that made me feel that I might be someone or something else separate as an individual was stripped away. After all, this is why I left home in the first place, wasn't it? Because I thought I was too good for something; I didn't know what, but there was a knowing that I wanted to do things on my own and live my own life. In boot camp, I was called "an individual" which was an insult because it implied that I was a person who would put my own needs first. Once again my individuality was repressed, and I would spend the next three months with strangers who dressed the same, acted the same, and looked the same as me. This was to become my new tribe.

The "psychological" training started at day one. I went through the first few days running from this place to that place, doing this and that, and I didn't even realize ... I hadn't slept in three days. The whole time we were all completely exhausted while running on adrenaline and hearing over and over that we are inferior. Inferior to real Marines, which we weren't yet. The physical routine was constantly changing so there was no way to "normalize" or "get used to" anything. While my brain was searching for normalcy, it would finally give in to the fact that there is none.

You never know what is expected. You surrender to following the next command without anticipation because you never know what the hell they want from you. When you are completely physically and emotionally exhausted, things build up, and break away just as quickly. You start to believe that everything that is being told to you is true, without even realizing it. There is a weakness in me and I am less than my version of my perfect self. In this mental state, I believed that I had to change to be good enough. Good enough to be a Marine and to go to war, this became my truth. After being broken down into nothing as an individual, the next part of my training began. Harmony! To act and think as a unit! This was one of the most powerful and possibly dangerous aspects of boot camp.

Now things finally became repetitive, movements you've learned, you now know by heart and are always performed the same way and at the same speed. And once you finally get it, it feels good. This is a refined "groupthink" where your group is now able to execute any command in perfect unison. This is the drill. You've learned to focus on the instructions of your leader and to gain harmony in your actions. You've learned the importance of individual action in teamwork is instrumental in the training of instant obedience to orders.

The largest obstacle I had to face was endurance. By enduring things like pushing my physical limitations and not knowing what's next, I was trained to overcome obstacles, like pain or fatigue, without question. I learned that, under extreme conditions, you can still run carrying all your gear with pain in your body and make it to the end. The discomfort doesn't stop you, you just keep running and somehow the pain goes away just as fast as if you stopped to cry about it. This mental training built a strength to survive. The much harder and longer training would further test me physically and mentally.

Isolation from the "Outside" Is where communication lines are nearly severed completely from friends and family for the most part. Except for the handwritten letters or the ability to make a phone call on Sundays. This was the reward for training well during the week. Otherwise, our training was never interrupted by distractions from the world outside of the one that is now being built.

For a few months, the Marine Corps became my entire world. I would experience what is known as the "Omnidirectional Ass Chewing" in which multiple drill instructors are just screaming at you in unison as you attempt to make sense of the universe around you. This experience will leave you frozen. I remember just standing there frozen, I could not decipher what was being said or by whom. My mind went into somewhere strange and I remember waiting for one thing. A clear command. Through all of this, I still felt this deep desire to be a part of something bigger. I wanted to belong to something and that something became the one person who was a constant source of encouragement through this transformation of my psyche.

M. Rene Harris

CHAPTER THREE

Still Small Voice

"Karma is the outcome of what you get when you defy the knowledge freely given you in exchange for the ignorance you hold as truth.." ~ M.Rene

During my three months of boot camp, my correspondence with Albert became deeper, meaningful, supportive and more loving. We talked about how he wanted to settle down with me. About marriage, kids, and a bright future together. After graduating boot camp, Albert and I would be married at my grandparents' home in Georgia. Two days before the wedding, his family and his best friend Seth came down from Michigan for the occasion. The day before the wedding, Seth and his wife took me out to lunch as sort of a bachelorette luncheon or so I thought. But it was just us, and they urged me not to marry him. I thought it was too late for that. I loved him and besides that, I'd already bought the dress and had the cake.

On the day of the wedding, while my mother was pinning up my hair and adjusting the back of my dress, I overheard a conversation going on around me.

"She doesn't look very happy," Albert's sister Terry whispered with her back to me.

"She's just nervous," his mother responded. To which his other sister Jessica replied, "Of course, she's just nervous." And gave me a wink.

My mother didn't say a word, she wasn't happy about any of this and I knew it. It was too soon for me to get married and she didn't feel this man was right for me. She'd told me more than once that she didn't like the way he treated me. She remembered the things that I had long forgotten. Things like me being stood up without as much as a call to explain. In my family's mind, he wasn't educated enough and he wouldn't be able to provide well for me. She hated the way he didn't care about what people thought but that was one of the things that I loved about him. I always thought that my mother was always huge on what other people thought. Appearances and keeping them up were how we had always lived. But now she couldn't seem to put her feelings aside for this one day. For me, I was getting married today. She finally relented and let me have the wedding but she refused to open her home to any of his family who flew in to merge these two families. I was appalled at my mother's behavior towards his family and apologized to them.

Later that day, I would overhear my mother say, "It won't last." It was then that I became determined to prove them all wrong. What I didn't realize in the ignorance of my youth is that karma would become defined for me in that moment. I would learn the definition of karma in years to come. Karma is the outcome of what you get when you defy the knowledge freely given to you in exchange for the ignorance you hold as truth.

As I walked down the makeshift aisle towards this man who would be my husband, I sensed the strong need to turn around and run. Walking slowly towards the pastor in my mother's living room was began to feel like walking through sludge. My legs felt as though they were heavy. I was tired. I was confused by what I was feeling inside me. "Am I ready for this?" I was now growing very concerned by the thing everyone said. I was supposed to do this, wasn't I? Everyone was already here, well almost everyone. I had spent nearly all the money I had earned from boot camp on this day and it seemed to be happening so quickly. Why did I want to turn around and run? Where was the backbone I had just found? Where was my strength, my pride? My sense of loyalty had now become my greatest weakness. I was walking towards danger and I felt it.

That night my father bought us a room at a nice nearby hotel for our wedding night. I was excited and nervous when we arrived. Not that we hadn't already been together, but because I was going to give myself to him as his wife and we hadn't been together since before I left for boot camp. It was going to be different tonight – I felt it. And different it was. Albert went straight to the mini bar and nearly cleared it out while he was on the phone with his long time ex-Army friend Dennis catching up on old times, a call which didn't end until long after I had given up and gone to bed and fell asleep from sheer exhaustion.

Early the next morning I got my wedding night sex, but it felt like every other time we had been together before. I had romanticized the moment, built up in my imagination what this moment would be like. Cuddles and kisses. Soft caresses while staring deeply into each other's eyes. But maybe that's not what it was supposed to be. I wondered what other people's wedding nights were like. Wasn't it was just supposed to be having fun with each other? I wondered if I had ruined everything because I didn't wait to give myself to him. The day next day would be spent with farewells to family and friends before packing up the car for our honeymoon road trip. The honeymoon was better than I had expected. We had a wonderful three days exploring the island. Making love with reckless abandon on the beach. Eating lobster dinners and best of all cuddles and kisses. Just like I had imagined it should be. Then it was time for me to report to the base nearby, for training. Since I had to live on base, Albert went back to Georgia and lived with my parents and secured his things while I surveyed off-base housing.

I found a small trailer in an even smaller trailer park near base as our first home together. It was cheap and soon after we moved in, it began slowly falling apart. Not only the small trailer, but our marriage was slowly falling apart right along with it. My sleeping patterns were lighter now. I would wake up as Albert would slip out of bed in the middle of the night, but I was so tired I would just go back to sleep and then wake up again when he would return home right before it was time for me to wake up. When I questioned where he was going or where he had been, he would say he couldn't sleep so he would just go down to the local bar that had a pool table and play pool or have a few drinks for a while. It had never dawned on me to question him or even check the time. We didn't have lots of time together so it didn't really bother me that he wanted to just go hang out and make friends.

Training days were long and sometimes overnight if we had field training. We would sit in a classroom for hours learning the ins and outs of what our jobs would be. I would work with classified files and spend most of my time in an office. When I wasn't in an office, I would be either in the field or hiking in full gear continuing to train my body and mind for eventual wartime. Near the end of my training, I received my orders and we were soon headed to my next duty station.

For the next two years, I began to notice that many of the women who were in my battalion were having babies. For the men, their wives were pregnant or had just had babies. My attention was starting to focus on why I was not getting pregnant. I am not sure why I wanted a baby, but it seemed like the next logical step.

I think it was a natural yearning to have someone to love and love me back that gave me a sudden sense of urgency to want a baby. Albert still wasn't working and still disappearing in the middle of the night. Maybe this is what was missing from our lives. Maybe what we needed to make us a real couple was to become a real family. After the third year of not getting pregnant, I knew something had to be wrong. Perhaps I wasn't looking clearly at what was really going wrong in my life at the moment. I wasn't looking at the signs. I had never bothered to ask the question of should I even have a baby with this man. I just knew that something needed to change and that change must be having a baby.

I made a doctor's appointment just to have things checked out. Was there a problem with me? Was having a baby even a possibility for me? It would take another two years to discover that the problem was, in fact, me. They took a small scope and went through my belly button to explore what was going on inside me. I had what was called endometriosis. My fallopian tubes were lined with scar tissue which could be preventing conception. It required surgery to go in and scrape the insides of my fallopian tubes and uterus because of the considerable amount of scar tissue that had grown. Albert was in the recovery room with me and had been told by the nurse that if he had anything he wanted to ask me and he wanted the truth now, during the time I was coming out of anesthesia, would be the time to ask me. I recall him asking me who my boyfriend was and if I had cheated on him. I informed him that I never cheated and I had no boyfriend, but I did apologize for killing his fish named Oscar. I also recall him showing up in my hospital room late on the next evening half drunk.

Returning home from my surgery, I hobbled up the steps to our second-story apartment, as the woman in the first-floor apartment opened her door and asked Albert if he wanted to come in for a beer. He quickly declined and followed me up the stairs into the apartment.

Later that evening, he decided that he was going to go out to the hot tub for a little while. I wasn't able to get the incision wet for a few days, so I lay on the couch to get some rest and watch a little TV along with some prescribed painkillers to keep the pain at bay. Albert got me comfortable on the couch then left to go down to the hot tub for a little bit while I rested. I fell asleep.

When I woke up, it was dark, a few hours had passed and Albert still wasn't home. I got up and hobbled my way down to the hot tub looking for him. There he was, still there, with the downstairs neighbor, the blonde who often invited him in for a beer when she thought I wasn't there. When they saw me, they immediately made a space between them and he invited me to join them and to go get my bathing suit and come on in. I felt a rage well up inside me, and instead of calling him a stupid mother fucker and throwing the plugged in CD player that they had sitting next to the hot tub INTO the hot tub, I quietly turned around and went back up to the apartment. Not only was I grieving at the thought that I was barren but now I felt unattractive and unwanted because of it.

I laid on the couch and cried myself to sleep. I told myself that he wouldn't have invited me if something was going on, but my intuition was nudging at me to believe differently. I ignored the warning signs firing inside of me and medicated myself and went back to sleep. It would be another hour or so before Albert would come home. After a few days of recovery, I was back at work on the military base. I was healing nicely and the pain was nearly gone. My days were long and it wore me out. By the time I got home, I was hurting and tired but still functional.

From the balcony of our apartment, you could almost see the hot tub and pool area of the complex. You could also see the service parking area behind the local grocery store. One night, while waiting for Albert to come home, I went out onto the balcony with a cup of coffee and a cigarette. I looked out at the lights of the small city neighboring the military base wondering when my husband would be coming home. I had prepared a nice candlelit dinner for us and the candles were starting to burn out.

As I stood on the balcony waiting, my eyes scanned my dark neighborhood dimly lit by streetlights. Then my eyes fixed on something in the parking area behind the grocery store. Was that Albert's car? I squinted to try and make out some detail but it was no use. I went inside and found the binoculars to get a better look. There he was, standing outside of the passenger door of his car. I couldn't get a good look at what he was doing. He seemed to be just standing there, on the outside of the passenger door facing the inside of the car with the car door open, but I couldn't get a clearer or closer view of anything more. I decided to put on my shoes and walk over there. I went to take one more look to make sure that not only was he still there - but to make sure that I wouldn't be approaching a stranger in the middle of the night. When I looked again - the car was gone. "Must not have been him after all", I thought to myself.

The next morning as Albert was taking me to work, I got into the passenger side of our car and noticed that there was a footprint on the windshield. A small left foot footprint. Made from the inside. The car suddenly stank like sex. I was fuming quietly all the way to work. Seething with fury. I didn't need binoculars to see what happened anymore. I was trying to search my mind for another explanation but I couldn't.

The next afternoon, my friend Emily came over because I was still very upset. My mind had run a million scenarios of what could have happened in our car. The conclusion always came out the same. As we were standing in the kitchen as I was telling her about what happened and just as the words "my car smelling like sex" came out of my mouth, I heard the front door close. A Short while later, Albert came in with a bouquet of flowers. Hug and kiss me and my temperature suddenly dropped. He had interrupted my thought pattern with the gift he had for me. He was being loving and kind and soft spoken. Albert had never brought me flowers before and my fury had nearly dissipated. This was the first time I had ever received flowers from any man. I had always wondered what that would feel like.

The following week, I again waited patiently for Albert to pick me up from work. I waited for over an hour and when he didn't show, my Staff Sergeant offered to take me home. I thanked her and told her that Albert must be working late.

We pulled into the complex and the car was parked in our assigned space.

"Maybe he just forgot?" she asked as she knew our car and saw the look on my face when I saw it too.

"I appreciate you going out of your way like this, I'll see you tomorrow," I replied while trying to force a smile. Maybe he just forgot.

I walked into the apartment and slammed the door; Albert rushed from the bedroom. "Hey babe," he said as he tried to usher me quickly into the bedroom telling me to get out of my uniform and into some comfortable clothes. As he was forcefully ushering me into the bedroom, I saw the patio door close out of the corner of my eye. He pushed me into the bedroom and closed the door on me, and when I was finally able to open it, I came out and went straight to the patio. I opened the door and no one was there. I heard a light click, I ran towards the front door and threw it open, I went out and looked down the stairs, no one was there. Then I turned to him.

Did I almost catch him with a woman in my home? I was so pissed at the thought of it I felt my blood boil. He stood there scared. I couldn't speak. I needed to tame my temper quickly, so I went to take a shower to calm down and to try to think rationally. I stepped under the hot water and took a few deep breaths. I wiped the water and the tears from my eyes and looked down. Thereon the shower floor was hair. Hair in my shower that was not his and it certainly wasn't mine. Long, dark, curly hair. This time, when the rage came, it came with a calm. I got out of the shower, dried myself, got dressed, and went in the bedroom. I took the first hard thing I could find, a small hard-topped Samsonite overnight carrier, the ones for makeup and small accessories, with the lift-out compartment on the top. I walked right up to him as he was standing in the small dining area just looking stupid and beat him with it. I hit him as he ran around the dining table trying to cover his head and as he ran for the door he yelled, "Who are you going to believe? Me or your lying eyes?" I ran towards him with a yell similar to a Samurai going in for the kill as he finally ran out the front door. I was too tired to chase him. I slammed the front door hoping he would stop somewhere and bleed to death. I sat down on the couch and cried so uncontrollably I was shaking. I cried myself to sleep on the couch only to be awakened by him coming in with his eyes red from crying, or so I thought. Albert curled up next to me and apologized for what I *thought* I had seen.

"It wasn't what it looked like," "No one was here" "The wind was blowing the doors, that's why you heard that sound" he began to explain. "Let's go away together, you need a break, you're just stressed out and overworked. C'mon, let's go to bed."

Maybe he was right. I was acting like an out of control crazy woman. We went to bed and for the first time in a long time, I fell asleep in his arms.

Things calmed down for a while but then a few weeks later, Albert would forget to pick me up, again and again, my Staff

Sergeant would offer to take me home. As she drove, she talked to me about getting my own car. Not that she minded taking me home but for my own convenience. We were stopped at a red light waiting to make the left turn that would lead us down the road to my apartment complex. As we sat at the red light, I happened to glance in the rearview mirror and there, right there, behind us was Albert. In our car with a woman sitting next to him.

I looked at my Staff Sergeant and remembered saying calmly, "I'll be right back." I got out of my Staff Sergeant's car and walked up to the passenger window of my car to where this woman was sitting ever so comfortable with my husband's hand caressing her inner left thigh. I went into what I can only describe as a blind rage, the window was down so I took the opportunity to pull her through it and began to beat her in the face. She lay on the ground trying to protect herself in shock from the attack that was happening to her right there on the side of the road.

My Staff Sergeant, Albert, and the young man and woman who were in the back seat quickly rushed to where this woman was on the receiving end of my entire wrath that didn't belong to her. Albert ran around the car and tried to grab me, but my rage turned quickly to him and I went straight for him swinging wildly, not landing a lick, as he continued to stepped backward to avoid my incoming swinging fists of fury.

My Staff Sergeant quickly grabbed me and escorted me back to her car, did a U-turn in the middle of traffic and took me back to the military base where I would have to meet with the Sergeant Major. I had committed a crime that day. I had attacked a civilian while in military uniform, in public. I knew my military career must be over as I waited in the chairs outside of the Sergeant Major's office while my Staff Sergeant went in to report what she had just witnessed. I did not feel remorse over what I had done. I was only ashamed of my behavior and at that moment vowed to never react that way again. The only words I remember Sergeant Major telling me were: "Well, I guess dynamite does come in small packages. Lance Corporal, you cannot fight in your military uniform. Don't ever let this happen again."

"Sir, yes Sir. Thank you, Sir"

My Staff Sargent took me home and Albert would return later that evening apologizing and explaining that it was again a misunderstanding. He was just giving those girls a ride to the beach. He went on to inform me that the woman was a friend of the girl who was in the back of the car with his friend John, who happened to be job seeking with him. I didn't believe any of it even though I wanted to. I wanted to believe that I had not made the huge mistake my gut was telling me I was making as I walked down the aisle on my wedding day. After much more discussion, Albert and I decided to go on a couples' retreat and renew our vows. It was a program that was offered by the local church for military couples who were struggling. I was struggling to feel hopeful throughout the weekend. I wanted so much to not fail in this marriage. I wanted to be a mother but I couldn't. I wanted to be wrong about everything. I wanted my mother to be wrong and for a minute I was feeling that I was on the right path until the last day of the retreat. We had finally worked through the getting-to-know-you and here's-what-I-appreciate-about-you stages of the retreat and the last event was the actual renewal of the vows ceremony. We stood there with several other couples and repeated the words of recommitment to each other, looking into each other's eyes as we repeated the promises. I was once again feeling hopeful until my husband said one final thing to me: "There, you happy now?"

I was crushed. I felt defeated and knew that all the things that had gone wrong so far were ultimately my own fault. I was a terrible wife. I couldn't give him a child. I was asking too much, I had unrealistic expectations. I needed to be better, give more.

Be more understanding. I needed to change but the sheer thought that another woman had been in my apartment was too much to wrap my head around so Albert and I moved a month later.

Somewhere in my mind, I reasoned that where we lived was part of the problem. But, in reality, everything else was the problem. Certainly, a change of residence was going to make things better. At least not staying in the same apartment where another woman had possibly been in my bed, in my shower, and possibly using my things would soothe my pain. Never giving thought to the fact that wherever I moved to, my problems were packing up and tagging along. They lived with me. I was married to them.

Months later, I was standing in front of the television in a dark, cigarette-smoke-filled living room, and another heated argument was full tilt. I was leaving him. I was yelling, but I can't remember what it was about this time because he stopped mid-argument and looked at me and said: "You're pregnant aren't you?" I froze and my brain shifted. "Why would he even say that?"

I wasn't supposed to be pregnant, where would he get that idea from? We had been married now for nearly four years and were told that our best option for children was to adopt only months earlier. I had given up hope of being a mother. This would be the worst possible time to be pregnant, and at this point, I didn't even want his child. And I certainly didn't want to be his wife anymore. I turned and left the living room without saying a word. I went to bed furious and decided that in the morning I would make a doctor's appointment just in case.

Early the next morning, I was in the garage which was located under our apartment. I was digging through papers and for the life of me, I can't remember what I was looking for when I found the stacks of porn. Then I looked on the workbench and saw these tiny crumbled pieces of aluminum foil and pieces of cut drinking straws. I couldn't figure out what he could have possibly been working on that would require straws and aluminum foil. I certainly knew what he needed the porn for and it hurt.

I opened one of the pieces of foil and saw a white powdery substance in it. Cocaine? That would kind of explain why he wasn't sleeping lately and why he was so cruel. He had changed so much. Was this why he was so unfeeling, mean, and careless. I was scared, it was like my hormones had flipped my "crazy" switch and I lost it. I ripped the pages from his magazines and taped the porn pictures to the walls on the garage and his car. If that's what he wanted to look at, let everybody look at it!

Talk about a fight! He was embarrassed but mostly angry. Not that I had found it, but that I had displayed it. I confronted him about the cocaine I had found. "You're so stupid, it's not cocaine, it's crystal meth," he said. With that, I was dumbfounded and left speechless. Mostly because I had no idea what crystal meth was, but I was now determined to find out. Maybe I had discovered our problem and it wasn't just me after all.

I began to research the subject. What was this stuff anyway? The more I learned, the more afraid I became. He displayed most of the symptoms I had read about on the internet: not sleeping for days, not eating, erratic behavior, and man, was he a mean motherfucker. I was now on a mission to heal him. I couldn't leave him now, he was sick and he needed me. Surely, this was our problem. He told me that he never wanted to be with someone who was sick. He had concluded that not being able to produce a child was some sort of sickness. He told me that he had always wanted to be a father and that my inability to give him children was the reason he had turned to drugs and other women.

My test results came back positive. I was pregnant and I was in complete and utter shock. My focus at the moment was not on being pregnant, it was on healing my husband and helping him overcome this disease. It wasn't until I began to show and my belly started to grow larger that I felt more fragile. More afraid. I would have nightmares and cower down to Albert easily now. Letting him come and go as he pleased for fear that I could not protect myself in my current state.

I was seven months pregnant when he first hit me. Slapped me right across my face because of something I had said that offended him. I threatened to leave him and he threatened me right back.

"If you leave, I will hunt you down like the dog you are, and you will never see that baby again," he seethed. I said nothing. I did nothing. I told no one.

I wanted to say "screw this" and just leave him but I couldn't; he was sick and I was pregnant and scared. The crystal meth had made him angry and violent. I can handle this, I thought. Maybe we can get through this together, after all, we had a child to consider. I felt a little hopeful about my decision to try. I would help him heal and save our marriage. Besides, where would I go? I'm very pregnant and I cannot defend myself. I was vulnerable and defenseless.

After doing some more research and talking to the Substance Abuse Counselor on base, I came home feeling determined. There was hope for families after substance abuse. Not often, but it does happen. I walked in, sat my things down and listened to the messages on our home answering machine. I stood there dumbfounded as I listened to the beginnings of a conversation that Mr. Dumb Ass had recorded between him and another woman he had been seeing.

"Hey babe, it's me," said the woman's voice. I heard him say "Hey" back with a little giggle before I ripped the phone from the wall and smashed the answering machine. Damn, I should have listened to the rest of that conversation but it was just enough to confirm that this wasn't going to work.

I knew that the decisions he was making were not logical. I knew it was because he wasn't right in the head and that he may never be. I knew that I'd need to make a new plan for my own life instead of staying. This wasn't going to work. He was never going to change. My new plan would be to re-enlist, get stationed in Italy or somewhere far away and take my child and never see him again. After all, he had threatened me and the baby, so my only hope was to take my child and run. Then fear gripped me in a way I cannot explain. I would not be able to move until after the birth of the baby. There was no physical abuse that I had reported and I was too ashamed to admit what was really going on in my home. So I would wait and while I waited, his mother came. She was going to stay with us and help out with the coming of the new baby.

During the time that she was there, he was the perfect, most attentive, most gentle husband ever. He was the man I always knew he could be. He had changed for the better. Was it just because his mother was there? Was it the baby that had made him open his eyes? His mother reassured me that he was a different man now and that he deserved a chance to prove it. He was sober now or at least I thought he was. I would not see him drink a drop for months. He was attentive and loving. We laughed together and he was tender for the first time in a long time and three months after giving birth to our first son, I was pregnant again.

His parents had offered us five acres of land to build a house on if we moved to Michigan. So after an extended enlistment while on active duty during Desert Storm and promises of sobriety and change from Albert, I declined reenlistment and a career as a Marine and became a reservist and at nearly eight months pregnant and with a baby on my hip, we drove across the country with all of our belongings to start our lives over again. To save him from going back on drugs. To save our marriage. To save his life. To save the lives of me and my babies.

Flies in My Coffee

4

CHAPTER FOUR

La Vida Loca

"Wherever you go, there you are." ~ *Jon Kabat-Zinn*

We lived with his parents for nearly three years before we began building what I thought would be a new home and a new life for me and our two young sons. His mother was one tough woman. She was a survivalist and knew how to do things that I had never even heard about in my sheltered life. She would often pick on me and tell me that vegetables don't grow in a can. She gardened and canned her own relishes, pickles, and tomatoes. She made a variety of soups and pasta sauces and other things like that. If she could grow it or pick it, it went into a Ball mason jar for later eating. I was amazed at her ability to do this. She bought in bulk, divided it and froze it, sometimes for years. She cooked things like squirrel and venison that people went out and killed on her property. This opened up a whole new world to me. There was more to surviving in this world than just keeping your feelings from being hurt.

She was active and resourceful. She attended the local church and was an active participant on a regular basis, but she was also as mean as a rattlesnake on top of all of that good work she was doing.

When the boys were old enough, I bought them a puppy. He was a small poodle mix his name was Brutus. He was warm and playful, and although we were forbidden from keeping her inside, the boys loved him and he brought much-needed happiness to us while we lived there. One morning, Brutus was at the back door in the garage, waiting for the boys to come out and play with him when Albert's mother came in from church. The solid door was open and through the glass door, I saw her come up the stairs and kick Brutus off of the landing and onto the garage floor. I went out after him to make sure he was going to be alright as he whimpered and howled at the pain that was inflicted upon him from this bitter old woman. That woman walked right by me with not as much as a word. This was her house and things were done her way and I learned quickly that the weaker would suffer for noncompliance. Brutus was hurt, not badly but just so that he wouldn't be hurt again or worse, I found a new home for him.

His father had been sober for quite a few years when I finally met him. He was kind to me even though he was outwardly cruel to his wife and grown children. He told me once that I wasn't "really" black. That I didn't act like a black person and I suppose that is what made me more acceptable. He had a brother who had shot himself in the head in his living room and Albert, who was still in elementary school at the time, found his body sitting in the La-Z-Boy. He also had another brother who was serving a life sentence in a prison in Virginia for murder, a hate crime which afforded him the opportunity to write a book while incarcerated. I knew very little about his family before but now I wish I had known all of this before I married him. This was now my children's family tree. Their lineage.

Who would my children become? Exactly what I encouraged them to be! I was determined to show them how to be better than what they were learning. But how? I wasn't even who I wanted to be yet and I had no idea how to get there.

Albert's father was his hero. He saw him as a strong and determined man, who had raised seven children on willpower and a fire in his belly. What he failed to see was the woman behind the man. The woman who stayed, took the abuse, birthed and raised the children in spite of him. To Albert, the roles were in proper order. To me, it was the ultimate dysfunction and a sadness that no one should ever have to choose to live with.

It was nearly 3 a.m. on a crisp fall morning, when Albert came staggering in, and his mother had awakened and came downstairs when she heard the noise. I got up and got him into bed, grabbed a bucket of water and a cloth to clean his vomit when she walked up to me and stopped me. She refused to let me clean up after him. She knew, she understood something. Later that day she would give me a book called "Codependent No More" by Melody Beattie. I devoured the book in no time. While I was busy taking care of a baby and a toddler, I had not realized that Albert had begun drinking again but it didn't come as a surprise.

As I read this book, I realized that many people had suffered from trying to love an addict. I began questioning this codependency thing, maybe it's normal to be codependent. It has to be. I hated the thought that I needed to be "recovering" from anything. After all, I wasn't the one with the problem here, he was. Living with his parents showed me that his mother had been "recovering" for a long time, while others, like me, are just beginning the road to recovery from codependency.

I didn't know what it meant to be recovering, or where this recovery would take me, but I knew I was going there anyway. I may be codependent now, but I damn sure was going to strive to be codependent no more. I felt that things would start getting better for us again if I set some boundaries and let him be in charge of his own recovery while I took charge of mine. That had to be good enough for now.

I pondered over what I read on a daily basis and started to recognize the patterns of addiction and what it did to the people whose lives were affected by it. Was I really enabling him, or was I protecting my children from seeing a shit show on a daily basis? Was it right to keep them from discovering who and what their father really was? While the process of recovery is learning to stop the pain, I saw it more as a light at the end of the tunnel.

I noticed Albert was drinking daily now, or maybe he always had been but I didn't realize it. His behavior now was different than I saw with the meth. He wasn't up for days and violent, but he was still mean and demeaning when he was around.

His father tried to encourage him to attend AA meetings with him occasionally. This only made Albert stay away from home more often. In his mind, he didn't have a problem, everyone else did. I began to pay closer attention to the interactions and conversations between his parents. His father was a bully to his mother. He would call her "holier than thou" and "stupid bitch" in front of my young boys. If she argued back on any level, he would say, "There you go! If I say it's white, you'll say it's black." He seemed to feel that any opinion she had was a direct confrontation with him somehow and maybe it was. But wasn't she entitled to her opinion? Wasn't she supposed to be able to see the world from her own eyes and not through his?

Later, like clockwork, I began to notice the conversations between Albert and I mimicking the same homogeneous characteristics of his parents. I would begin to hear the exact same words as if they were a written script. I had heard them before, but until now, I had no idea where they had come from.

I witnessed the daily, and exhausting, back and forth between his parents, and I began to ask myself "Why doesn't she leave him?" and "when is enough, enough"? One night, I lay in bed praying, asking God the same question: "When is enough, enough?" As I began to fall asleep I heard a quiet voice say, "Enough is enough when you no longer tolerate that which is intolerable." I woke up the next morning with that phrase still in the forefront of my thoughts. These words would repeat themselves with nearly every interaction I had with Albert. They would ring like bells in my ears when I witnessed his father degrade his mother. These words would be the introduction I needed to start my journey of questioning everything happening around me. I didn't want my children to grow up thinking that this was some kind of normal. It wasn't normal, it wasn't what I wanted as their version of normal. This was not the example of family that I wanted for them.

I stopped questioning Alberts drinking, I stopped caring if he did or not, and stopped cleaning up his vomit. I stopped worrying where he was when he was out. I stopped praying for his safety. This seemed to somehow put a fire under his ass. He became motivated to start the building of our house. The house developed quickly once we got started. We worked together and spent all of our time together. I learned to lay tile, run wires, connect plumbing, level a board, and pound nails (who knew that there was a method to that?). As the house got closer to being ready to get its certificate of occupancy, I had all but forgotten that I was recovering from anything. We were getting along now; he would have a beer from time to time but nothing major. We moved in before the house was completely done, but at least we were out of his parents' house. Even though they were just a short hike through a wooded trail, we were finally in our own home.

It wasn't long before Albert let me know that under no uncertain terms was this house being built for me. The house was to be used as a model so that he could start building other houses like it. I needed to keep clean at all times for showing. I kind of understood that and told myself that I could live with what I believed to be the beginnings of growing a financial future, a profitable career for my husband and a happy family. I felt a glimmer of hope again as I settled for this arrangement. I felt that I could somehow make this house a nice home for our family in spite of the fact that it wasn't mine. Things just may be starting to look up if I didn't expect so much. If I could just show him, just prove to him that somehow his family deserved it.

Albert began working as a carpenter and I tried to help grow his side company while he worked for a local builder. Sometimes he did a few side jobs on his own to keep food on the table and pay the mortgage. A year later, the house was still unfinished. We had kitchen cabinets with no drawers and bathroom floors with no tile, only plywood. The kids would get splinters in their feet after a bath if I didn't put something down to cover the wood. People would joke and say a builder's house is never finished, like a cobbler's family never has shoes or a plumber's house never has plumbing.

I guess that's possible, but it felt like just extreme laziness to me. In my mind, we just weren't important enough to see anything through to completion. And what about all the people that were supposed to be coming to look at this "staged" house so that you could show off your skills? What about them, where are they? They never came.

He wasn't bringing in much money, which I found odd because he "worked" all the time. But still, work was work and carpentry was hard, physical work. I tried to encourage him as much as I could when he complained about the work not being there or not paying enough. It didn't take long before he began the descent into his old patterns. Soon, he would not show up at work for days, and I would get phone calls from people he worked with looking for him. Most times, I had not seen him either and thought he was working.

I was growing angry and my anger made me afraid. For my children's sake, I needed to find solace in something. In order to be present for them, I needed something to avert the fear, confusion, and anger that was starting to grip me. He was becoming even more controlling. When my sisters would call, if he was there, he would act out in ways that made it nearly impossible to have a decent conversation. I didn't want them hearing him yell at me and it wasn't in the background either, he would make sure he was in the same room, if I went into another room to talk, he would follow me. He would comment on my portion of the conversation or start yelling about something as stupid as me not watching the spaghetti boil. I would learn to talk to my family when he wasn't home. Eventually, the phone calls from my family got fewer and farther in between.

He didn't want me watching soap operas because he didn't want me getting any *ideas* in my head. I loved *All My Children*, I had followed the show for years. I would try to watch it while the boys napped, but soon, I would lose interest in that too. I was losing interest in everything. His mother would come over and go through our things in the disguise of "cleaning", rearrange my furniture, and then go and tell her friends from her church that my boys were little demons. People would see me in the local grocery store and laugh about how she talked about my children. I would smile and laugh with them. I am sure she may have been kidding, but inside my feelings were hurt. I was feeling the familiarity of isolation. I needed a tribe. I needed community. I finally found a local church in the next town over. Maybe it is spiritual guidance, prayer, and worship was what I was lacking in my life.

I was struggling to feel love for my husband. I found it harder and harder to forgive him for little things. I was starting to see him as less than what I hoped a husband should be. After he would say or do something hurtful, he would complete the action or words with "You hate me now, don't cha?" I would ask

him not to say that to me. I didn't want to hate him. After years of hearing that, I was starting to feel it and it was growing stronger.
I delved into the church, into the Bible I had since 6th grade.

I found a church that I really liked and that only seemed to make him angrier. I desperately needed to feel acceptance. But it seemed the more active I got in church, the more I prayed, and the calmer I felt, the angrier he became, the nastier he was. Until he decided to start going to church with me.

M. Rene Harris

CHAPTER FIVE

Faith and Scars

"God will not look you over for medals, degrees or diplomas but for scars." ~ *Elbert Hubbard*

Church became my new tribe and our new battle ground. I wanted to go to church, I needed it. It made me feel good to belong to something. I grew up in church, for the most part, and it was something familiar. Besides, I had nowhere else to turn and I was looking for salvation. I was in a crisis internally and I was seeking comfort. At first, I started taking the kids to church with me alone, while Albert stayed at home.

It wasn't as welcoming as I had imagined it would be. I think I had this image that I would be welcomed with open arms by all of the congregation. Inviting me with hugs and warm looks of compassion, as if a lost sister had found her way home again. The church was mid-sized, full and cold. I would find a space in the back and sit and try to keep the kids seated for an hour while I listened to the message.

Over time, I would find myself sitting closer and closer towards the front and eventually I was invited to have my boys attend the children's services. Finally, I didn't have to spend the entire time trying to get them to sit still and not disturb the people around me who were trying to hear the message that was delivered that day.

When Albert decided he was going to go to church with us, I was shocked, then I became excited. I felt hopeful that my prayers were being heard and that God was answering them. It didn't take very long before church became something else to argue about. Another tool in his tool belt that he could use to deconstruct any form of belief that I was gaining through my new found community. Maybe this was the Devil trying to challenge the work that God was trying to do in my marriage? I was taught to believe, in a subliminal way, that whenever you are trying to do something good or whenever you are trying to live right, that the Devil had nothing better to do than to try and stop you. This battle between God and the Devil over anything good that we strive for would be something that many religions are taught to live with.

Apparently, the Devil had nothing better to do than torture people who were coming into their natural calling to walk in unison with the Creator. Even though it didn't make sense to me, I came to want to believe it to be a truth. The truth that somewhere, somehow, there was a being equal to God, fighting for my thoughts and behavior. Fighting for the outcome of my actions through fear and manipulation. The thought that somehow we were not responsible for our lives. That If something was not going right, the Devil was responsible. It seemed foolish to me to give the Devil more power through the energy of fear than we offer to an omniscient God who happened to the creator of everything including the Devil.

I would tread through my days with this duality in my spirit, but there was a bigger nudging inside of me. I knew there had to be a higher truth out there. I tried to believe that God and the Devil were in a fight for my very soul. I would pretend to live it, but I would not be able to let this settle as truth in my gut. What I was feeling went against everything I had been taught in growing up. However, for now, I concluded that this must be the way to my salvation.

We arrived on Sunday mornings appearing like the perfect family. I felt haggard and exhausted from the battle that would take place on the 30-minute drive just to get there, only to want to not even be there when I got there. The ride home was often another 30-minute argument over why he didn't believe in the message that was delivered that day. Maybe it was his attempt to have a healthy debate about religion or the message itself, but I felt it was a means to tear apart my beliefs. Inside, I was still without a unit, without her tribe, and before long, the whole church experience would become exhausting mentally and spiritually. I was unable to wrap my mind around the contrast between debate and command, argument versus demand. Between honoring what I knew inside and believing what I was told to be true.

To me, he was attacking my beliefs and that would torment my mind. I sought solace in the only thing I had learned to know, silence and withdrawal. Inside I was struggling, I wanted to submit to my husband, to follow him but how could I follow a man going nowhere. I was trapped in my own world of confusion.

Albert promoted himself to the church as the leader of the home. A firm believer and a great father and husband, and to my utter amazement, they believed him. He attended a couple of men's events and it actually looked like he was really getting involved as well. But when he returned home he was unchanged, unrepentant, and callous in his unbelief. So much that he would begin to tell me that God didn't care about me. He found the perfect opportunity to insert that I was "holier than thou" in any conversation that had me give my own opinion on any subject. One Sunday, I mustered up the courage to go to the pastor of the church for prayer. I wanted my husband to be "saved and filled with the spirit of God" I told him. I was called a liar. I was told that he knew my husband and he was "saved" and "filled with the Holy Spirit." They noticed he comes to church and sits in the front row every Sunday. They all noticed how he held the baby while he was sitting there, they even noticed that when the Pastor would demand the congregation to hold up your Bible if you believe every word of it is true. Sure it was noticed that he didn't do it but that was because he couldn't, he was holding the baby. And when the Pastor would ask the congregation to stand if they believed the message. Sure it was noticed that he didn't do it but that was because he couldn't, he was holding the baby

I told them that he didn't do it because he didn't believe any of it and that he had told me as much. To my surprise, Albert had told them that I was the non-believer and I was crushed. Crushed that a Man of God would stand in my face and call me a liar for asking for prayer, and crushed that Albert had worked his way into deceiving the church to believe that he was something he swore he didn't believe in. Didn't they hear from God? Didn't God tell these kinds of Holy men what was true and what wasn't? Was my husband a Christian? But wasn't I the one who was there helping clean the church? Helping with programs and events? Was I redeemed or was I just out of place in my role as a wife? The words from my husband's mouth, "God doesn't care about you," "God doesn't hear your prayers," and "God doesn't want you praying about little things" would ring in my head. I couldn't believe that. I needed to believe that God heard me, that He cared about my pain, that He cared if I was here. Was God even there anymore? Was the battle over my soul a waste of time so much so that God didn't even want it anymore?

I stopped going to church, and I began seeking the answers on my own. I needed to hear from God for myself. I needed to know what was true. My spirit was broken. My heart was broken. I needed to end this mental battle before I lost my mind. God was going to speak to me, and I wasn't going to stop seeking Him until He did!

It was a sunny afternoon when I received the phone call that my mother had been diagnosed with breast cancer. Albert drove me and the kids to Chicago so that I could somehow help my mother and father during her chemotherapy sessions. The distraction of caring for my mom and trying to be there for her helped to distract me from what I was going through back home.

I tried very hard to assist my mother and father during this difficult time while also caring for my young children and trying to keep them out of the way. Things were beginning to take a strange turn that I didn't understand. With the devastating reality that a cancer diagnosis brings and in my mother's attempt to get healthier, she asked me to take away her cigarettes, hide them, and not give them back to her even if she asked for them, even if she yelled at me and I agreed. I was so proud of her. I felt useful and I had a mission. It felt good to be helpful, to be needed for a greater purpose. It was less than 24 hours when she asked for her cigarettes back, and when I refused to give them to her just as she asked and she became furious. She got so mad that she had my dad tell me to give her back her cigarettes.

"Whose side are you on anyway?" I asked him.

"I'm on the right side, now give your mom back her cigarettes!" he demanded.

"I will not!" For the first time in my life, I was defiant to one of my parents. It was a scary but empowering feeling. I was doing a good thing; I couldn't abort my mission now. I thought maybe I would be commended for my convictions, but I wasn't.

A week later, my mother would ask me to leave. Well, she told my father to tell me to leave. I was devastated. I was so hurt, and I didn't understand why my punishment was so severe. I was only trying to help as my mother asked me to. My father was apologetic, but my mom wanted me gone. I called Albert, and he drove to take me and the kids back home. Shortly after we returned home, I would receive a letter from my father that would shake my entire world. He wrote apologizing for my mother kicking me out when he knew I was there to help. He wrote that my mother was angry and felt that my father and I were lovers and had been since I was a child. That is why she really wanted me out.

I cannot remember ever having cried so hard. It felt like an episode of the Twilight Zone. I could not fathom how my own mother could conceive the idea that my father and I were lovers, which in itself is gross. But if she did, why kick me out? If she felt that something had happened to me as a child, why not protect me? Why turn her hate to me, a child, her child? Albert's mother read the letter; some compassionate part of her saw my pain and she wanted to take the letter and destroyed it. I was numb. "You don't need to be reading this garbage," she told me.

I shared what my dad had written with my sister, who shared it with my other sisters, and we had a conversation on the phone with my mom about it. I took that opportunity to ask my mom the one burning question I had.

"If you thought someone was hurting me like that, why didn't you protect me?" I asked her.

"I thought I was protecting you. That's why I sent you to live with your sister when you were twelve," she said. Out of the eight of us, I was always the black sheep of the family. I knew I wasn't my mother's favorite by any means. But I never knew, until that moment, why she sent me away. She had always made that clear in how she treated me that I was not her favorite. I wasn't my father's favorite either. Dad treated me the same as all the other kids. He was always working and really too busy to show any of us any special attention.

That was the answer? That's how she handled her daughter possibly being violated by her father? She sent ME away? I kept calm and assured my mother that Dad had never in any way done anything inappropriate to me. My sisters assured her as well, but I don't think she was convinced. I hung up feeling that I was alone in this world, but finally understanding the hatred that my mother seemed to display towards me.

I still had to function somehow. I pushed the whole thing inside of a tiny box inside of me where I kept all of my bad memories. I could not deal with this, or any of the other fucked up ways I was seeing my world right now. It was too big for me, too heavy. I had my children to raise and a crazy husband to deal with right now. It would be a long time before I spoke with my mother again.

I would wait for Albert to leave for work, tend to the kids and get them off to school, and then it was my time to seek God. I devoured my Bible, every chapter, every verse. Praying and asking. Questioning and crying out. Seeking some sort of truth. Then one day, answers began to come, but not in any way that I had ever expected. Something had changed and to this day I couldn't put it into words if I tried. Albert became somewhat non-essential. He was no longer much of a focus. I didn't hate him, but I didn't love him either. At least, not how I felt I was supposed to love him. I was no longer having dreams of him chasing me and trying to kill me. I no longer dreamed that I was trying to protect myself from him. My dreams were different now.

I had always had premonition types of dreams. From a small girl, I knew there were messages in my dreams. Dreams so vivid, so real, so colorful, that I could not forget them. Dreams so powerful that it even changed my behavior at times. But now my dreams were different. I recognized that they had enormous meaning, and I would start to learn to pay very close attention to them.

My dreams had answers to many of my questions and showed me direction but they also showed me other things. Months after the letter from my father and the conversation with my mother, I had a dream that my aunt had come to visit me. She would not come in the house but would stay outside. She wanted to take a look around the backyard. I went outside where she waited and I showed her around.

"Why did you come here?" I finally asked her in the dream.

"I told your mother that I would come and say goodbye" was her reply.

The next morning, I received a phone call that my aunt had passed away that same night. I would not go home to attend her funeral. Then the dreams stopped. I prayed harder but the more I tried to communicate with God, the more I felt he was just up there twiddling his thumbs, creating earthquakes, arguing with the sun to rise and shine, making thunderstorms, but only in places that didn't need the rain. Was he ignoring me?

I delved deeper into seeking God on my own. By myself, in secret. In the privacy of my own room. My spirit knew there was something more and kept drawing me to continue to search. The dreams would start to come with messages that only later I would begin to understand.

One day I had taken the kids out to the local library when I stumbled upon a curious book. It was large with gold-colored binding. It stood out to me, so I grabbed it and began to look at it. It was a Hebrew-Greek Bible with literal English translation. It had three columns, each column written in different colors. So I took it home and began comparing it to the King James' version of the Bible I had grown up with. I had studied Theology and Religion for a semester in high school but I was no expert on the subject. This seemed the perfect complement. Exactly what I was looking for. I was enthralled and amazed at the contrast. Truths that I had not known before seemed to jump off the pages at me.

These words, these truths, agreed with me on some level. I knew my Bible, or at least I knew what I was taught to believe about it. But I had no idea of the secrets that lay within the pages of this book that had become my lifeline. I needed God to prove himself to me. Was everything I was taught to believe wrong? I wanted the truth to show up big in my life before I made any decisions about ending my marriage. The thought of divorce, in itself, would mean failure to me. It would mean that I gave up, surrendered, and threw in the towel without giving God the chance to help me.

One night, I dreamt that there was a tornado coming up through my backyard, but it wasn't my house, it was my mother's. I was standing at the back patio door. The storm was dark and the funnel was coming towards the house quickly. However, I was not afraid, I was sad in this dream. My children and I would be able to take cover in some kind of cellar, but the tornado would touch my mother and all of her things would be caught up in the winds of the storm. Three months later, I received a call to come home, that my mother was very sick. I didn't hesitate to pack up and go to her. She is my mother. Maybe this is my opportunity to finally make things right. I felt like I had spent my entire life trying to get my mother's approval. Even through my rebellious stages. I needed her love and once again she needed me and I would go. No questions asked.

I would spend two weeks caring for her and taking her back and forth to the hospital. Her cancer had returned, and this time, it had metastasized throughout her body. The doctors had put a timeline on her life. My sisters arrived and hospice had been called in to help. My mother would die in her home and in my arms. I don't remember crying that much at that moment. I felt I should have been distraught throughout the day but I wasn't. I was sad, very sad but my sadness and grief didn't deter me from being rational. There were things that needed to be done. Details that needed to be addressed and someone had to be strong. That someone was usually me because I had a way of turning my emotions completely off and getting done what needed to be done.

That night, my grief found me and I silently cried myself to sleep on her sofa. I dreamed that my mother had come to talk to me. She sat next to me on her sofa and I told her I was sorry. She told me that it wasn't my fault and that she had a gift for me. She looked pretty, she looked healthy and happy. Not the way I had seen her earlier that day – frail and small.

She then told me to look in her closet in a green purse and I would find it there. The next morning, I got up early and went for a run around my parents' home. There were giant magnolia trees in bloom and the beauty felt so overwhelming I began to cry. I don't know how far I ran but I was too emotionally drained to run back, so I walked slowly and thought about my mother's last 24 hours. "I should have called 911. I shouldn't have given her that pill. Why didn't I just call 911?" My mother had a Do Not Resuscitate order. She was ready to go, but it was the most difficult decision not to try. Not to do CPR or call for help as I watched the life slip from her body and she took her last breath. I let her go. I let my mother die without doing anything.

My mind was racing even though, last night, in my dreams, my mother came to comfort me. When I got back to the house, I went into my mother's closet, located the green purse up on the shelf and looked inside. There was a small digital Bible in it. I knew that was what she intended. I felt a presence and turned around. My father stood there in the closet doorway and told me to take everything in my mother's closet that I could fit in. He wanted me and my sisters to have it all. My sisters and my dad had decided that I should have my mother's mink coat. They wanted me to have it for taking care of Mom. I took the coat and held it as if I was holding my mother, one last time.

After the funeral, Albert, me, and the kids drove back home to Michigan. It was a good two-day drive, and we were tired the evening we arrived. The kids had fallen asleep in the car, and Albert and I didn't talk much as the radio was playing and served as a distraction for any real communication. We arrived and went in the house to put the kids to bed and retired for the night ourselves. Before I could get too rested with my eyes shut, one of the noisier toys in the house had started to make noise. I sighed and got up, thinking one of the boys had gotten out of bed and was playing with the toys. I walked into the living room intending to see one of the kids sitting there wide awake and ready to play, but no one was there. The noise had stopped. The toys were piled in the middle of the living room floor, exactly the way they were when we left. I went to check on the boys in their room, and they were in bed, sound asleep. As I walked from the boys' room and across the living – there was a toy truck, a larger Fisher Price or Tonka type that the boys could sit on and scoot around with their feet. The kind that made various noises when you pushed random buttons. It was separated from the other toys. Was it there a few minutes ago? Maybe I was just sleepy. I started to walk very slowly through the living room when suddenly that truck started to make random musical noises. No one song played to completion – it was as if the buttons were being pushed randomly as the songs changed. I grabbed the toy to turn it off. It was already off. I took the batteries out and just stood there looking at it – and waiting. I closed my eyes and whispered to my mother's spirit. "I don't want to play. I want to go to sleep." I went to bed and started to fall asleep thinking, "I'm throwing that thing out in the trash tomorrow."

More dreams came, they came fast and clear and surreal. My search for God turned more metaphysical and I could feel my spiritual life growing. One thought began to run constantly through my mind. One of us had to do something to change the direction of this life we were living.

Flies in My Coffee

CHAPTER SIX

Bad to Worse

"I have done something wrong, something so huge I can't even see it, something that's drowning me." ~ Margaret Atwood

Anytime I wanted anything extra I would be reminded that I needed a job. We needed things. Things like better food and nicer diapers. I was able to secure Medicaid, food stamps, and WIC from the state, but I was ashamed that I had to turn to state assistance. I had a husband who was fully capable of working and he should be providing for us. He was only five years older than me, and at 33 years old, he was still pretty healthy physically. There was no reason, that I could see, that we needed to go the route of welfare. I had urged him at one point to go work for Ford Motor Company. His father had retired from there and he had two brothers-in-laws who still worked for the company. It would have been so easy for him to get a job there, and it was a good, stable company that would allow him to provide well for his family. He refused.

Our son John was chronically ill. He was constantly in and out of the hospital with respiratory issues. He was constantly being treated for pneumonia or bronchitis and was regularly taking antibiotics, until one day on a visit to the doctor, I was told that he was faking it for attention. I knew in my gut that something was wrong with my child and could not accept this as a diagnosis. With John being sick all the time and only four years old, I couldn't go to work yet. I needed to be at home with him.

After the ridiculous diagnosis, I searched and found a new pediatrician, one closer to our home. She was new in town, and when I went to see her, I felt an immediate connection. She was listening to me. Finally, someone was listening to me and I trusted her. She requested his medical history and researched his symptoms and found that he may have actually ingested amniotic fluid during his birth. Since it had been years of improper diagnoses and treatment, his lungs were now failing. Just before John's 5th birthday, he had gone into respiratory arrest and was taken by ambulance down to U of M Children's Hospital in Ann Arbor, Michigan.

When they got him there, they ran several tests and prepared him for surgery on his lungs. He had a hardening in his bronchial tubes that they could not remove. The hardening was killing the healthy tissue that could not get oxygen to it. After the first surgery to chip out some of the hardenings, they moved him to a private room for observation. While my baby lay in the hospital bed, a kind nurse came in. She had a glow about her. She told me that her shift was over. "The doctor will be coming in the morning, but for tonight – he has been given all of the medication that he needs. Do not, under any circumstance let anyone give him anything else. Do you understand, Mom?" I agreed and she left.

A few nurses came in throughout the night to check his temperature and his blood pressure. It seemed like they came in every hour or so. At 2 a.m., a nurse came in; she looked small and frail, and her frame seemed to have a dull dark shadow surrounding her. I felt like I was dreaming as I lay in the hospital bed next to my son trying to get a little bit of sleep. She said she had been ordered to give him an injection of something, I couldn't quite understand her.

"I was told that I am not to let anyone give him anything," I told her.

"Ma'am, the doctor ordered this for your son," she argued with me.

"I don't care; you are not giving him anything and you need to leave," I stated.

She was frustrated with me as she started flipping through her chart again. She prepared the syringe on a stainless steel table next to his bed, and I got up from my bed and stood in front of her between her and my son's bed. She stepped back and quickly flipped through her medical chart again and left. I sat on my son's bed, exhausted. I looked at him, watching him sleep. I kissed his forehead and stroked his hair, wondering if I had just made a big mistake. A few minutes later, the nurse came back in, but she looked different. Perhaps it's because I was awake now.

"Ma'am, I apologize. I went and spoke to my supervisor, the head nurse, and sure enough, if I had given this to your son, it would have probably sent him into cardiac arrest. You are one smart lady to watch out for your son. I don't know how this mistake was made. I am so sorry," she told me.

I was too tired to say anything, it all seemed like a dream. She left the room with everything she had brought in and apologized again as she stepped out. It all felt like a dream, but the dark shadow was gone. I never saw her again, nor did I see the kind nurse who warned me. I still think she was an angel or something because when I went to find her the next day, to thank her, no one knew who she was. The doctor came in around 9 a.m. They never come at 7 a.m. like they promise. He explained to me that they would need to remove the lower portion of my son's right lung where the bronchiectasis was located in order to save the healthy tissue.

That did not sit well with me. I needed to consult with his doctor first and I refused to allow them to perform the surgery. somehow I knew something higher was happening, I couldn't explain it. I didn't "feel" it - I "knew" it. Unquestionably. The report had gone back to his doctor; she was understanding and tried to explain to me that the tissue they could remove would help him, but that, of course, there were cautions and precautions that we would have to take if we chose this path. I decided to think about it and I did. The surgery would be risky and could lead to more damage.

During the next month, I went into something that I can only describe as a type of prayer with determination mode. I visualized my son healed. I visualized him coughing up whatever that was stuck in his lungs, but in my visions, it was black and thick.

I sat in the kitchen drinking a cup of coffee and reading when John started coughing. It had been a little more than a month since his hospital stay. The cough from him brought all of my senses to full attention, it always did. I prepared his nebulizer treatment with systematic and autopilot-type movements. We had done this several times before. I set up his video game on the television in front of the couch to distract him. Grabbing a clean mask, tubes, tissues, and a juice box, I poured the liquid into the machine and placed the mask over his nose and mouth, but this time, he was fighting me. He couldn't breathe he was coughing so hard. The cough was thick and wet. He had tears in his eyes. He choked and gagged as this thick mucus began trying to come up out of him. I immediately turned his fragile little body down on my lap and began to perform what we called percussions. This is when I would cup my hands and gently "play

Bongos" on his chest and back. Almost like patting someone on the back when they are coughing to force air into the lungs.

The goal was to make it easier for him to expel the mucus in his airways, which in turn should make it easier for him to breathe.

He coughed and gagged aggressively. I tried to remain calm in order not to alarm him as he looked up at me with his large hazel eyes with fear. I told him it would be okay, that I had him. I turned him over and grabbed some tissue and began clearing his throat of the mucus. I used Kleenex to physically pull the thick mucus from the back of his throat. The more I pulled from his mouth, the more he gagged and fought me. The mucus was thick, but unlike my visions, it was clear at first, then yellowish, and the more I removed, the more he coughed and the darker it became. I ran and grabbed a washcloth because the Kleenex was sticking to his tongue, and pulled more of it out, just off the back of his tongue.

I wanted to stop and dial 911, but I couldn't stop now and let him just choke. "Keep coughing, baby," I told him; as long as he was coughing he was breathing. But then he stopped. He stopped breathing and in a panic I heard myself scream, "Come out of him now!"

And with that command, this black chunk of what I could only best describe as tar came out of his mouth. He started coughing again but just a few times and it was different. It was dry and weak. He was breathing. Breathing normally. He was tired and his little body was weak. I knew in that instant; my son was healed.

I called the doctor's office and made an appointment to see her at her earliest availability. I didn't feel the need to rush to an emergency room or call her over. It would be a few days until we could get in. She called from her home and asked me if everything was okay. I told her yes and I told her what happened. She said she would see me in a couple of days, but if he started coughing again, forgo the breathing treatment and take him to the nearest emergency room. He didn't cough anymore, and the day of his appointment, we got dressed and went into her office.

"I would like him to have another x-ray," I told her.

"You know what we're going to find, he just had an x-ray a couple of months ago," she replied.

"I know, but I would like him to have one anyway, please. I think it's gone" I said.

"He really doesn't need one, but if you insist, and because he had the episode you described, we can go ahead and do it anyway."

"I insist." I pleaded.

We headed down for x-rays and I sat and waiting for his x-rays to develop. He hadn't coughed since that day. I knew something had happened, I just felt it. We went called back into the examining room where she asked me to tell her what happened again a few days ago. I told her again.

"I want to show you something," she said as she walked me into the hallway the led to her examination rooms. On the wall was a large framed board that was illuminated in order to see x-rays clearly. Two sets of x-rays were clipped on the board. "You see this? This is John's last set of x-rays. You see that dark area down here? This is where the problem was. Okay, now look at this." She pointed to the set of x-rays that she had just taken. "These are his lungs today. See this area right here?" She pointed to an area on the x-ray. "This is where we would normally find the same thing as we did over here," she said as she pointed to the old x-ray images again.

"There is nothing there, do you see that?" she asked with wonder in her voice. Tears rolled uncontrollably down my face. There was nothing in his lungs anymore. It was gone. "I can only describe this as a miracle,"

.

I went home and packed up all of his medical equipment. We wouldn't be needing that anymore. But we would need to find a climate that his lungs could continue to thrive in; the cold air of Michigan in the winter would not help him stay healthy. Where would we go? How was I even going to leave? I needed my husband and what little money he was bringing in or at least that is what I believed.

It felt humiliating asking my husband for money for the things that I needed. I had asked Albert for money so that I could buy tampons or Kotex. He simply told me no. "I only need five dollars," I plead with him. He just looked at me and walked away. I learned to use rolled up toilet paper or washcloths as feminine items. I needed a job so that I could buy my own damn Kotex. I couldn't take care of myself as a grown woman. My pride was crushed. My self-esteem had long gone but to beg for money just to have basic necessities, served as a vital lesson in my need for independence. I wanted to depend on him to take care of me. I wanted so badly for him to provide for my basic needs but he couldn't. He wouldn't.

I finally got a started working part time at a small local clothing store. I worked there for a few months and I loved it until my niece got really sick. She was on life support and the family was called to come together. When I told my boss that I couldn't come in for my shift because a family member was imminent, I was told that if I left, I should not return. We were short staffed, it was inventory time and I had the closing shift. I ended the conversation with my supervisor with a "Thank you for the opportunity". I decided it was best to continue to stay at home with the boys until they were a little older. Time seemed to fly by and the boys were now in 2nd and 3rd grade. I would try once again to venture into the workforce. I landed a job working full time for the State in my first management position.

I worked for nearly a year, traveling from Senior Center to Senior Center within the northeast counties. I was planning menu's and visiting homebound clients. Not really managing any people but my title said Manager none the less.

The job required some traveling and my only concern was the care of my children after school until I got home. I did my best to make it home by the time they returned from school but often I wasn't able to even get into my town before dark. I finally got myself a car and was beginning to feel pretty good about myself. I felt a little sense of pride and a little increase in my self-esteem. I had heard that people do things more to avoid pain than they do to gain pleasure. I suppose that's true because I think I worked more as a distraction, a way to stay away from home, more than I did for the satisfaction of work.

I drove many miles across the state in many road conditions. From white outs in winter blizzards to hard rains in the spring. But it was a dry, clear and sunny day when I was leaving the main office in Alpena when I was in a car accident. I was about to turn on a small street headed to a nearby Senior Center when a truck sped out of a shopping center parking lot and hit me head on.

Everything went black.

I remember the ambulance and one of the EMT's inside of my driver's side door trying to remove me from the car. I remember bits and pieces of a conversation. I remember struggling against his effort to remove my top in order to listen to my heart with his stethoscope. I remember hearing, "Hold her still.". as I struggled to get off the gurney and get back into my car so that I could go home. I remember thinking "Albert's going to be pissed."

My next memory was lying on a stretcher with a brace on my neck. I remember hearing someone say "She's in shock" as I tried to get up off the stretcher and pull my blouse together.

I remember the bump of the stretcher being pulled into the back of the ambulance. I remember thinking "I don't have time for this". The next thing I remember was being at home.

For nearly two weeks after the accident, I was doing physical therapy and resting at home while waiting to be released back to work. After a couple of days, I was becoming restless. It was on a beautiful Saturday morning and the leaves had begun to turn their auburn color and were starting to fall from the trees. If you have ever been to the Midwest in the fall then you know the beauty of falling leaves when they blanket the ground in their rich hues of reds and orange.

I woke with my body still a little sore from the accident but it's not too bad today. The kids were still sleeping and it was the perfect time to clean the kitchen and sit with a cup of coffee in the morning quiet. After a while, I decided to go out to try to do some work in my yard for a while. I was attempting to rake up some leaves out front when I saw a car pass by for what seemed like the second time. This time, he stopped near a house up the road. I noticed that the man in the car was taking pictures. He seemed to be taking pictures of me. I stopped what I was doing and went inside not knowing who this creepy fellow was. I would later discover that he was from an insurance company and that act of raking my yard for a few minutes out of boredom would later cost me my job.

After a few of months of no income, my car payment lapsed and my car was repossessed. I watched as they hitched it up to a tow truck in the middle of the night. It didn't take long before I fell into a deep depression again.

I was so close to self-sustainability but now I was trapped, again. It felt like I was absent from myself. I felt sad all the time. I was robotic in my day to day life, like a zombie, void of the capacity to think or feel. And once again I would discover that I was pregnant.

I was depressed. I struggled to get out of bed and shower. I struggle to get the boys off to school, prepare dinner, and things like that. I had found myself avoiding being touched by Albert. I couldn't even look at him as if the fault alone was his. My search for meaning had ceased. I was mad at God. How could He let this happen? Why wasn't He doing something? Now here I am, pregnant and useless, for the third time.

I did it anyway and I reasoned it away by making myself a victim to his empty threats. He would say things like "I'll beat the kids" or "If I don't use it, I'll lose it" or start random stupid fights that only the act of sex would end. Did I do it just to keep the peace? Or did I subconsciously want affection so bad that I needed the connection from him? There was no real love, or emotion, although when I gave my body to him I felt my heart trying desperately to reach his. It made me physically sick at times. It made me cry every time. John was already 7, nearly maintenance free and my life was just beginning to feel like I could get on my feet. Like I could just grab that door handle and open up to my perfect future. Life on my own with two kids would not be easy, but now there are three. The thought was overwhelming. How was I supposed to get a job and run away with two elementary school aged kids and a baby? I felt like I got the "Go back to Start" card.

The depression had gotten to the point where I was now prescribed antidepressants during the pregnancy. I was maneuvering each day on autopilot. Directionless… hopeless. My children would be my motivation to live, but in order to really live, I would need more than motivation than not to die. I needed a reason for being alive. I don't recall much during that time, but I did know that I needed to get my shit together if I wanted anything in my life to change, anything at all. I began searching harder and more fervently than ever before for something higher. Something higher than me. Something higher than the God I knew.

It was Father's Day weekend and the boys now 8 and 9 years old recognized the day with excitement. Steven, the baby boy was almost 2 years old. Anything that excited his big brothers excited him as well. Over the weekend, I told them I would help them make gifts from construction paper to give their father on Sunday. When the two older boys got home from school that Friday, we put our creative hats on and went to work. We had glue, stickers, crayons, and glitter for our tools as we constructed paper houses with brightly colored animals and cars for him. We would not see him that night. When he came home late Saturday afternoon, he was drunk. John was so proud and excited that he grabbed his gift and ran to him before I could stop him from approaching his father in the kitchen.

"Daddy, look what I made you for Father's Day!" John squealed excitedly.

"Does it look like Father's Day to you!?" Albert snapped. He grabbed his well-constructed gift and threw it at him. The sadness in my son's eyes is a look that I will never forget, but a look that I would see more often than I would care to admit. As John began to cry, his father told him to grow up. I grabbed my 8-year-old and hugged him, whispering in his ear that I was so sorry and that everything would be alright. I was disgusted with this man and his cruelty.

I had heard about meditation and decided to try it, or at least try to quiet my mind from the incredibly negative chatter that was consuming me. All I knew about meditation was that I was supposed to sit cross-legged, put my hands on my knees and be quiet. I had no idea what to do next. So I sat there, thinking.

Reviewing the past seven years in what seemed to almost be like a movie playing in the front of my mind. I guess I thought that my mind was supposed to calm down and do something different. I didn't know what the "different" was supposed to be. I just knew it was supposed to be different.

Over the next few months, I would put the baby down for his naps and I would go and sit, crossed-legged, and just think. Then it hit me: I'm not doing this right. I needed to find out how to do this right. So back to the library, I went to find books on how to do this meditation thing the right way. The more I read, the more I learned that there is as much about the subject of meditation as there was about anything else. There were also as many versions of what meditation was and how to do it as there were books in the library. Like colors of a spectrum, the versions seemed endless. I needed one way, the right way, and I somehow needed it to be an end-all be-all fix that I could understand.

I needed my "Ah-Ha" moment. But the more I studied, the more questions would present themselves to me. Questions that needed answers. Answers that I didn't have and that I couldn't seem to find. I wasn't giving up on my search for God, in fact, my search had widened to find truth by any means necessary. By this time, I realized, that the Bible I had grown up with, seemed to have been taken out of context so much that I could hardly listen to any preacher without picking apart the message they were attempting to bring.

I sat listening to messages streaming through my television from various televangelists and compared them to the scriptures. Cross-referencing their messages in order to find the true meaning. I discovered through the Greek and Hebrew versions of the scriptures, that many had been distorted in translated. Truth had become slanted in such a way that religion itself seemed like a fairytale to me. One with no end, some with no hope unless you believed the fragmented stories. Without blind faith, there is no hope for miracles, financial blessings, or any of the other gifts Divinity was holding back from us until we either get it right or gave enough. I began to delve into the study of Buddhism in my attempt to find peace. It seemed to be where peace came from. I wanted to know more about this thing called "Enlightenment".

Nearly a year had passed, and it was Albert's birthday and the boys wanted to bake a cake.

"Can we make Dad a cake for his birthday?" they asked excitedly.
"What kind of cake would you like to make?" I asked them.
"Chocolate! Chocolate cake with chocolate frosting!" they squealed. So we baked a cake. The boys helped mix the ingredients; they loved cracking the eggs, but licking the bowl was the best part of any childhood baking time.

We watched *The Fox and The Hound* for what seemed like the millionth time while the cake baked in the oven. After the movie and the cake had cooled down, it was frosting time. They gently spread the frosting over the cake, the plate, and each other. Placing the candles in the exact right spot was important for Clark, so that was his job. We laughed for what seemed like the first time in a long time.

Then we waited for their dad to come home. He didn't.

The next morning while the boys were having breakfast, Albert came stumbling through the front door.

"Happy Birthday, Dad!" roared the boys. I looked at him with what must have been such a seething rage that if he could have been incinerated at that moment, he would have. He walked into the kitchen, stood at the unfinished island in our unfinished kitchen, and stared at the cake.

Flies in My Coffee

"We made you a cake, Dad," John said, smiling up at his father.

"You made this?" Albert asked.

"Yup, can we sing happy birthday now?" Clark smiled.

Without an answer, without hesitation, and without a thank you, Albert stuck his full hand into the cake, squished it in his fist and shoved it in his mouth. "My favorite kind is German chocolate," he said as he scraped the rest of the cake into the sink and went to bed. I was too tired to cry, too weak to fight, and too numb to do or say anything. I felt like a coward. I was a coward; I was weak, I was useless.

My tolerance was coming to a breaking point. I knew that if I didn't do something that I would die just like this. Weak and voiceless while life continued to pass me by. The problem was that I didn't know what to do or how to do it.

Spring came and went and the warmth of summer was wasted on my days shut up in the house. On this particular day, the boys played outside in the dirt and sprayed each other with the hose until dinner time. After a bath and a Disney movie, the boys fell sound asleep but I still couldn't sleep. It was late, around 1 a.m., and I couldn't sleep. Albert wasn't home so I lay on the couch watching TV. Flipping through the channels, I stopped on an infomercial that I had seen before but never really paid attention to, but this time, it was different. I was paying attention.

There was a man with a large face talking about how I could live an extraordinary life. That I could discover the power of greatness within me. He wasn't a televangelist, but he was passionate and pretty convincing. It would cost money that I didn't have to buy this tape program, only $99.95, but I wanted it so bad. When you have nothing, a hundred bucks seems like an enormous amount of money.

I wanted to change my life; I needed to know how to change my life. I wrote down the information and waited for Albert to earn enough money before I could start to siphon small amounts at a time without his knowing. Once I had stashed away enough I called and finally purchased the Anthony Robbins' tape set on how to change my life. After all, it was refundable. And if it was a scam, if it didn't work, at least there may be some secret message locked inside that might help me get headed in the right direction.

Flies in My Coffee

CHAPTER SEVEN

Failure to Thrive

"A fool's paradise is a wise man's hell." ~ *Thomas Fuller*

Albert's sister, Sarah, and her husband Josh were visiting from downstate. They sat down and talked with me and Albert about the roles of the man and wife in a relationship. Josh had tried to convince Albert to take a job with Ford Motors down in Detroit, and Albert was still very adamant about not working there. His reasons didn't make sense to anyone. He didn't want a socially acceptable job just because that was what society expected of him. Josh went on to explain the benefits that it offered him and his family, but Albert didn't care. He felt that by doing his own thing, he provided well enough for his family. He felt that we didn't need any of those things.

"But Albert, you even have retirement and life insurance in case anything ever happened to you," Josh told him.

"I'm not getting any life insurance! If anything happens to me she can pay my debts when I'm gone," he snorted.

It looks like I need to get a job, but when I do this time it's going to be a good one, I thought to myself.

I knew at this point that I needed more than just a job; I needed a career. I needed a way to provide for myself and kids that would make a good life for us. If I was going to leave this man, I needed to be strategic: just packing up my three boys and leaving wasn't an immediate answer. It didn't have to be. He reminded me several times over the years that at least he wasn't beating me, and true enough, he wasn't physically beating me. But emotionally, I was battered and bruised. Steven was almost three years old and old enough to be left with a babysitter so that I could work again. One morning after getting the big boys off to school, I grabbed the local paper from my in-laws and while Steven played with toys that had no batteries, I enjoyed my cup of coffee and began looking for a job.

I saw an ad in the paper for a position at a new hotel. This was perfect! I used my mother-in-law's car to drive over to the hotel to apply. It was beautiful and I knew I had found something special. I was eager during my interview. They were looking for help in the spa and although I had no experience, I convinced the Director that I could learn. I was hired and I learned fast. I absorbed every bit of information I could about the hotel and the spa that was available to me. I helped the Director with everything from researching products to writing procedures for her. When all of the initial opening duties were complete, I maintained the spa receptionist position and answered phones, booked appointments and cashed people out after their services.

One night I was at the reception desk of the spa, running my reports, and closing down for the day when Albert called. He was drunk. I was trying to tell him that I couldn't talk, my boss was right next to me, but he kept on. He was yelling now, telling me that his life was worthless, and threatening to kill himself. My boss was overhearing my side of the conversation. She could see that I was upset but offered nothing in support.

She went into her office which was still less than 20 feet away from the reception desk and sat at her desk pretending to do some work. She left her door open and listened to what seemed like was the longest conversation of my life at the moment. I told him I would be home soon and we could talk about it. I was actually more concerned about losing my job than I was about him killing himself. My shift ended and I rushed home hoping to find him dead. He wasn't there when I arrived; he would come home at nearly sunrise, throwing up in the front yard, walking past me, and passing out in the bed. The next day, I went to work and was written up for taking personal phone calls during business hours. At least she didn't fire me.

I worked very hard but made very few friends simply because I didn't have time for it. I was on a mission. I went in, did my job, and went home to be with my kids to act as a shield from the drunken onslaught of verbal garbage that would be thrown at all of us by their father.

Another year had quickly passed and I needed a challenge. I applied and was promoted to manager in a different department of the hotel. It was more money, but it required much more time away from home. I finally began to make friends at work, I began to feel a little more normal. A little bit stronger.

But at home, things were starting to become a little bit worse.

It would be another year later and I would be promoted again but this time as the director of the spa department. I felt inadequate for such a position. I felt like I had no idea what I was doing, but I kept telling myself that I could it. I could find the answers, I had to do this. I will do this. I had no choice. Sink or swim became my motto. I was making more money than I had ever made before; it wasn't a lot, but it was a salary and it was helping. It was just enough to make us ineligible for any more state assistance but only enough to pay the bills and cover food and other necessities without much extra. I had benefits like medical and dental insurance. I felt so grateful and determined to make this job work.

One day, I was called to the desk by one of my receptionists who had become frustrated while speaking with a customer. This particular woman was very wealthy and eccentric. She often made appointments but rarely came in for her treatments. She was canceling again, and I found myself compromising with her.

"Rebecca, if you come in this time, I'll throw in an extra upgrade for you," I told her.

"I don't care about that; I'll pay the cancellation fees if that's what the problem is," she replied.

"That's not the problem at all," I told her. "We just want to see you. But if you don't show up this time, I'm afraid we won't be able to make any more appointments for you. You will have to just show up and if we have something available, we will take you."

To my surprise, she showed up, with tuna fish sandwiches for me that she had made. She swore that she made the best tuna, and she did. Rebecca and I would become fast friends. She would invite me to her home, which was on the water, and quite beautiful, yet unfinished. I told her that my husband was a carpenter, and she should have him give her a bid to finish the upstairs portion of her house. Rebecca and I were talking on the phone one day and she told me that she needed a new car. She had a Lincoln Navigator that was too big for her and that she wanted something smaller, something sportier. I had no idea what a Lincoln Navigator was and I really didn't care until she said, "You should take my car and I'll just get a new one."

"I can't take your car, Rebecca. I can't afford a car like that," I told her.

"I'm giving it to you," she replied.

I was floored! What was going on here? This woman cannot just give me a car. Wouldn't that make me obligated to her on some level? Something didn't feel quite right about being given a car, much less a Lincoln Navigator, by this eccentric rich woman who obviously didn't have a lot of friends.

This was a sketchy situation and I couldn't put my finger on exactly what it was that was happening here. Was Lady Luck finally on my side like this, or was this a situation I needed to be cautious about? The best way to deal with this was to agree to pay something, anything, just so that I would not feel under any obligation to this woman.

I called Rebecca and offered to pay her $100 a month for the car. I told her that I could not afford more at the time, but that I wanted to pay something and not take advantage of her kindness. She agreed, and the next week, we went to pick up her new sports car and she signed over the title of the Lincoln Navigator to me. A few months later, I would introduce Albert to Rebecca and he would agree to become her personal construction worker by finishing her loft and building her a beachside pool-house. I would continue to pay her as agreed until something felt very wrong.

It was our anniversary, and Albert had not come home last night. It didn't really matter, though. But when Albert did finally decide to come home the next afternoon, he brought me flowers in a vase and gave them to me.

A lovely bouquet of wilted lilies that I recognized from Rebecca's dining room table only days before when I visited her home. While I was there, she invited me to enjoy her hot tub and began to tell me how her new "boyfriend" kept praising her breasts as "the perfect breasts." She must have made this statement at least three times, and I never responded because, well, how do you respond to that? I didn't want to see them so what was the point? Then it hit me.

If this woman rarely left her house and was ashamed of how she looked because her teeth, which were literally rotting out of her mouth, when did she find a boyfriend? She would make dentist appointments and not go to them. She was an eccentric trust fund baby and was squandering away her portion of her inherited wealth on drugs and extravagance. When I visited her home, she would proudly show me the work that my husband had done on her projects.

After a final visit to her home, along with the stories of her new boyfriend, I paid closer attention to what was being offered to me by way of information. There was little progress on the construction and I realized that her new boyfriend must be my husband. I had my suspicions, but I was so fixed on my plan of leaving him that I didn't even bother to address it. The information added to my list of evidence as to why I should leave. I couldn't be distracted from my goal. Not now. I did not have time for a breakdown and that's exactly what would happen if I let my feeling get in the way. I couldn't let this get the best of me right now. I suppressed and stuffed my emotions further down in the back of my mind so that I could try to stay focused on my goal.

Rebecca called to invite me for a visit to have lunch in her home to which I firmly declined. I stopped taking her phone calls after telling her and my husband that he could work off the value of the vehicle from now on. She would not get another dime from me. After all, he wasn't bringing home much more than weed anyway, and that didn't serve me because I don't smoke.

The Navigator was starting to display electrical failures and other issues, and I kept having to schedule appointments to take it in for repairs and the cost was adding up. So, since I owned the vehicle free and clear and I needed to be free from any attachment to this woman clear, I traded it in.

It was the beginning of a beautiful summer weekend. The kids were out of school for the summer and I would stay at the resort with the children and my niece who had come to help me out, like a live-in sitter situation. We were having an event at the resort that weekend and staying on the property was perfect and very kind of my General Manager to let me do.

My niece being there as a nanny was the perfect situation. I needed to work, but I also needed a sitter and she was a girl with a gypsy spirit who needed a place to rest for a while. The boys loved her and she was great with them. She was young, creative, loving, and active – everything I couldn't be to them at the time. I tried to reach Albert all weekend, but I couldn't. The boys wanted to talk to him.

Albert wasn't answering his phone or returning any messages. I knew that he had planned to attend an outdoor music festival that weekend while the kids and I were gone, so I tried not to worry about him as I went on about my business helping with the event. After the weekend was over, we returned home. He was there as if everything was normal. I believed that he had stopped seeing Rebecca months ago. He wasn't leaving the house at all hours or taking private phone calls. Lyndsey began calling me insisting on payment resolution and I told her what she could do with her payments. Albert was being nice again, giving me attention and complimenting me regularly on my appearance, which I was severely self-conscious about. It was the middle of a beautiful afternoon and my niece had taken the kids out to the beach for the day when Albert and I found ourselves at home alone.

I was starting to feeling pretty good about myself, my job, and the atmosphere was just right. Albert had walked up to me and from behind, his hands caressed my arms. He held me tight around my waist and began kissing my neck. I didn't reject his advances, on the contrary, in that moment, I was his. He wanted me and I needed to be wanted. Exhausted and sweaty, we laid there at the end of the bed, and with a smiled and looked into those piercing blue eyes once again. It seemed like years since I had felt what I was feeling. Was I feeling love for him again? He looked back at me and as I searched his eyes for meaning and connection he told me what he had done that weekend. He told me that I needed to go and have myself checked because one night at the festival, he had sex with a woman he didn't know.

He was calm and unrepentant as he told me the graphic details about how she was high, she was in a tent, and that several other men had enjoyed her as well. He said that she didn't mind, she was young, maybe a college student or something, and that she had large breasts. Then after questioning him, he told me that he did not use a condom. He told me that she wanted it and that she was cool with it. But he said the good thing was that he couldn't have an orgasm because he felt kind of guilty.

I was in shock and could not speak. I lay there naked as my mind searched for solid ground as this rug had been pulled from under me yet again. The casualness in which he told me all the details about what happened was crushing. He told me how he had already gone to the clinic and gotten antibiotics because it felt like he had BBs rolling up and down his penis. The image of BBs from a BB gun came to my head. I had to get a visual to understand what he was saying to me. He told me that he was waiting for the test results to come back, but he felt that maybe it was all in his mind because of the guilt.

After I could breathe again, I began crying so hard I was hyperventilating. I asked him if he thought what he had done to this poor girl was rape. If she was under the influence, then she was not fully aware or capable of knowing what was happening to her. Shouldn't he have protected her from being gang raped by these strange men instead of being one of them?

Shouldn't he have done something more heroic? But, of course, I was being self-righteous right now, he said. "Holier than thou" and judgmental. My mind could not wrap itself around what was happening, what I was hearing come out of this man's mouth. Then he would finally say again, "She asked for it, she was okay with it." I told him to leave.

I screamed at him to get out.

He told me he wasn't going anywhere.

He finally left and went to his mother's house for the rest of the day. I cannot describe with enough words how I felt. My brain was lost in a sea of confusion. Every emotion imaginable raced through my being all at once it seemed. The kids would be home soon and this too, I would have to set aside and deal with later so shut the door on my emotions and tended to my children until I could get to bed and cry myself to sleep.

The next night, I told him I wanted to go to the local bar and have a few drinks so we could talk. He agreed. When we got there, we ordered a beer and I grabbed his pack of cigarettes from across the table and lit one. He asked me please not to do that. I had not had a cigarette in several years.

I told him that I wanted him to leave, that I wanted a divorce. He said he talked to his mom about it and she told him not to leave. That we should go to counseling again. He was demanding counseling at his mother's suggestion. However, he had conditions for this counseling before I even agreed. Ok so first of all, I'm the one you cheated on in such a grotesque way and secondly, I'm the one asking for a divorce; so how is it that this man thinks he can put demands on anything to make me stay? Am I missing something? Surely I must be. He continued listing his conditions and I listened.

The counselor would have to be female, first off, and she could not be affiliated with the church in any way. I agreed because I figured this would be a safe way to be heard and leave without too much of a fight. I would later discover that it was his mother who had instructed him not to leave because it would look like abandonment to the court system.

The next morning, his mother came over to visit, more like her regular control visits. She told me that Albert had told her that he had an "affair" and that the only reason he did it was because I stopped communicating with him. I just stared at her.

"I can't do this" is what came out of my mouth out loud.

"Yes, you can," was her response. She had no idea that I was referring to having this conversation with her of all people.

"Stay for the kids, these kinds of things happen, this too shall pass," she said. This was her motivational speech to me after only hearing his side of the story? Of course, it was! Why should I expect anything different?

I agreed to go to marriage counseling but for the purpose of having someone in authority convince him that this marriage was a bust. I wanted him to come to the realization that we were just no good together. I went in with no intention of staying with him. On our first visit, when asked if we were there to try to stay together or to separate amicably. He quickly answered that we were trying to stay together. I quietly answered that I wanted to separate.

It didn't take long before he began to tell the story of what a horrible wife I was. How I didn't clean under the dishwasher. Yes, "under" the dishwasher. It never crossed my mind to clean "under" the dishwasher. He told of how his mother did our laundry, which she did when we weren't home without asking my permission. He told of how I was never satisfied and was seeking business venture after business venture, which was absolutely true.

It was our third or fourth counseling session when I concluded that the marriage seemed more like a slavery attempt than a partnership and that his drinking was causing behavior that was unhealthy and dangerous. He encouraged to seek out a 12-step program like Alcoholics Anonymous. When it was suggested to show love in a caring and understanding manner, he blew up stating that no one had right to tell him that he didn't love me or how to show it.

He never returned, and I continued the counseling on my own. The last day that I saw her, I was continuing to complain about him and his wrong doings when I was faced with my own inability to identify my self-worth. I wasn't ready to hear that my narrow perception could be skewed. I had such a distorted view of my perspective that I could not dis-identify with my limited perspective. I was so absorbed in my limited perspective that I could not clearly and objectively see my own shadow.

I almost forgot that I was supposed to be making a new life plan and now that I wasn't going to therapy I was encouraged to go back to trying to create that plan. Over the next few months, I would commit myself to my life changing audio tape series. There were workbooks and step-by-step instructions on building a better life. An extraordinary life. A life that, if I could imagine it, I could live it. Each day there was a lesson and homework.

On the weekends, there was either an interview or a subliminal recording to listen to. I could start to see life in a different way. I was making a plan, and this time, I knew what I wanted for nearly every area of my life. This was so doable that I could almost taste it. Steven was in kindergarten when I took the steps to look for a higher paying job and started a job search. I needed a better job in order to have the life I wanted for us.

I wanted to go places and see things with my kids. I wanted things that I never knew I wanted before. I could do this. I knew I could. I had been on interviews in Atlanta and Florida, but that was not where I wanted to be. With the advice of John's doctor, it was decided that we would need to live in a climate with drier weather, someplace to live for the health of his lungs. So that summer, I decided to focus on Orange County, California. It was dry, warm and would also give me the opportunity to grow my career. It also had cleaner air than LA but ultimately, California seemed like a dream come true and that is where my focus and intention was now turned.

Before I knew it, another year had gone by and I consciously tried to work on the vision of what the rest of my life could look like. It took a lot of effort and daydreaming in order for me to visualize the possibility of a new chapter of my life. I knew what I didn't want, that was the easy part. But in order to translate what I didn't want into what I did want, it would take more mental work than I realized. It would take hope, faith, and belief in order to change my focus from not wanting to wanting. I had to know what I wanted and that it was possible that I could have it.

The tapes encouraged me to change my thinking from the negative and focusing on what I knew I did not want to thinking positive and focusing on those things that I did want. In other words, if I didn't want to hurt, I would have to focus on feeling good. But not only that, I needed to discover what made me feel good. This had become a foreign concept to me after being in survival mode for so long. My dreams were still strange and surreal. I dreamed that I was either running from him, leaving him or trying to kill him with a spoon. One particular night I dreamed of a red, white, and blue-nosed plane that crashed into a glass building, then another would crash only one wing through a smaller building next to it killing all those who were inside. I was inside the building, watching the wing of the plane as it sliced through the wall of glass windows of my office. I was somehow able to make it down to the streets and watch the shards of glass fall to the ground. When I looked up, I saw the head of a bull in the sky, larger than the sun. Tears of blood poured from its eyes and I heard the word "war." I was terrified, believing that this dream meant something significant. It was on a Sunday morning in June of 2001 when I went again to the Pastor of the church and told him about it. I didn't know who to tell but I felt it so significant that I needed to tell someone. The Pastor called the leaders into a meeting and had me tell the dream again to all of them. They had decided it didn't mean anything. I was not convinced. This was three months before the tragedy of 9-11.

Shortly after that, I remember dreaming that we were in the church that we used to attend, the same church that dismissed my needs and called me a liar. It was praise and worship time and the music was playing. We were singing and I stopped. I looked up and I saw water coming down from the back wall of the altar almost like a light trickling waterfall. Then the water got heavier and heavier.

I stopped and looked around, surprised that no one seemed to notice what was happening except me. Everyone was still singing and dancing, with their hands in the air in song and worship. As the water started to rush down the wall, it tore violently into the platform where the musicians played their music, and where the podium stood to wait for the Pastor to begin delivering his message. The force of the water pushed everything from the altar and into the pews, the musical instruments, and the people. The water rushed up one side of the wall of the church before becoming a giant wave that expelled everything and everyone out of the church doors and onto the street. My feet were barely wet as I walked through the damage and mangled bodies holding my children's hands. It would be another few months before the Pastor was injured in a terrible accident of some kind. He had broken his neck. I was becoming afraid of the premonition type dreams that I was having and people were becoming afraid of me. Those who weren't wanted to know if I could either see their future or interpret their dreams.

The hotel I worked for was transitioning into a high-end luxury hotel chain. We worked long hours in order to prepare and learn how to be part of this new brand. In an effort to expand my social life and gain support, I began hanging out with some of the girls from work for Girls Night Out once a month. During this time, Albert would call while I was out and threaten that he would beat the kids if I didn't come home soon. I felt the threats were idle but annoying and embarrassing enough for me to comply with his demands. In order to keep the peace, I would let him have sex with me every now and then. I would hold out until the arguments started getting really bad, then give in by backing my ass up towards him and letting him do his business until he was finished. It felt dirty and gross. I would wear sweats and granny panties to bed so that he was not encouraged. I went and had myself tested regularly, which was humiliating and was prescribed antibiotics even though nothing major was found just in case. But it eased my mind.

It was early February and the flu was already spreading. I was feeling sick and stayed sick longer than usual. I thought that maybe it was because of the high stress and long hours. By the spring when I was still sick, Albert looked at me and said those God-awful words to me: "You're pregnant, aren't you?" There was no way I could be. I had a surgery when Steven was a baby that removed a tumor so large that it took my right ovary and fallopian tube, part of the back of my uterus and a portion of my bowels.

According to the doctor, some cells don't behave and simply grow out of control and turn into nothing but a mass, and this is what happened to me. I had asked for a total hysterectomy at that time. I was never planning to have any more children, but the doctor advised against it. He didn't want to force me into an early menopause. "Besides, the tube and ovary that we are leaving are so damaged, chances are that you will not be able to conceive again."

I was five months pregnant when I had my first OB/GYN visit. I was distraught. But I figured as long as it's not a girl, I could handle it. I remembered a dream that I had when I was 12 years old. I was divorced and had four boys. I was in my mother's old kitchen, sitting in a dining chair and my boys were tall and standing behind me.

This must be my 4th son. A month later, I would discover it was a girl, and a month after that, I would be ordered to bed rest. I tried to work during that time anyway because the company only gave 90 days for FMLA (the Family and Medical Leave Act), but I had trouble walking.

In my final weeks, I was forced to stay on bed rest. My daughter had just been born when my 90 days were up. I tried to go back to work, but it had only been a week and I was still bleeding. I was released from my job.

My job search continued and the new baby was only four months old when my new life would begin.

Flies in My Coffee

CHAPTER EIGHT

Voice Lessons

"My heart was not broken over him: it was breaking for the things I had wanted from him. And I didn't want them anymore."
~ Rebecca Kelk

I had completed my new life workbook. I took the time to do the work and write down all of the things that I could imagine for the different segments of my life. The financial, physical, career, social, and family aspects.

Once I got a clear picture of what I wanted in these aspects, I was challenged to write out, in clear detail, what these aspects of my life could look like if I could have it any way that I wanted. If I could see it, I could have it. This is what the program promised. Soon I would be invited to interview with the management company that posted a position in California.

The hotel hired a management company that in turn hired me and placed me in a particular hotel. When I agreed to take the job, I was instructed by this management company that no matter what my paycheck said, no matter what company signed my paycheck, that I worked for them. I thought that was a strange thing to say to someone but okay, whatever.

It was clear to me that their intention was to eventually manage all of this company's spas, and that I was their ticket into the contract with this mega-hotelier. If they could place me in this position and have the management contract, I could somehow convince the ownership to let them manage other properties that had spas. Maybe it was because I had 9 years' experience and my position had covered more than one property, so I was a prime candidate to show what they brought to the table as a management company. It seemed devious and sneaky, but I accepted the job with my eyes and ears open. I wanted this job so badly. The salary was three times what I was making and they would relocate me and my family to California. My plan was unfolding right in front of me. I accepted the agreement and was hired.

We drove from Michigan to California for this new opportunity. As part of the relocation package, we were able to live in the hotel until I secured other living arrangements for my family. We lived in the hotel for nearly three months before we found a large, beautiful four-bedroom, two-story house in San Juan Capistrano. Because the job opportunity happened so quickly, Albert would be responsible for putting the house in Michigan up for sale. My mission was made very clear by the General Manager, in a very short time. Either the spa made money or he could see no reason to keep me. The honeymoon was definitely over, and I needed to figure out fast how I could do this. Being the new girl at work was over already, and I would have to prove myself quickly.

The operations were eating up any revenue the department made. There was no profit and the staff ran the place. It felt like watching a scene from a movie where the prisoners had taken over the cell block and no one knew how to control them.

I blended quickly with the other department managers and my staff and I made friends rather quickly. In the first couple of months, the Vice President of the management company that placed me at the hotel would make regular visits to meet with me. We would review where I thought the opportunities for growth for my department were. He would ask me what I thought could be done and ask me to make a report. Then he would take this report to the General Manager and I would later discover that he would pose this report as his own ideas.

Over the next couple of months, I would see the billing from the Management Company on my P&L reports, which would have been fine, if they had actually done any work. I would eventually meet with the General Manager, Harold of the hotel and go over these charges that I didn't quite understand. I was combing carefully through my profit and loss statements when I saw that I was being charged for flights, food, room nights, and other travel expenses.

The problem was that after two months there had been no more visits, only random phone calls. They had been charging me for these travel expenses plus their monthly management fee of $2,400 for months when I discovered the "error."

"How can you make more money in the spa?" Harold asked me.

"I can save you $2,400 a month immediately if you fire that management company," I replied.

"But don't you need them? Look at the reports, they have some good ideas," he said.

"I will forward you my notes and emails. Those are my ideas and they have not been here in three months, but they are still charging you for their travel expenses."

Harold's face turned red. He was angry and he had every right to be. He sent the 30-day notice to dismiss the management company, and at the time, I didn't realize that I could be burning the bridge to grow my career by firing this company. I didn't care; I would build my own bridge. I felt that I could do anything. That anything was possible. I was passionate about growing this spa, about seeing it successful. I was on fire.

Over the next year, I would reach out to local women's groups, create a custom scent, and place the product in the guest rooms to cross promote my department. Our revenue exploded and in less than a year, I would take my department from loss to profit and I was a superstar. I was invited to attend owner's dinners and give presentations. The owner's representative was now calling me directly to ask questions, to check in, and ask how things were going. I was being courted by product vendors – lots of them. I had the power to say yes or no to any product that would grace the shelves of my spa and I took that very seriously.

But with every up, there is a down, and while I was busy creating avenues of revenue to grow my department, the hotel was being investigated by the Labor Board, and I would unknowingly be right in the middle of it as a key witness.

The Wedding planner was a very attractive, and flamboyant man named Kevin, who had contracted HIV. He confided to the Director of Human Resources and was fired. Big mistake. The Director of Human Resources had told his story, all about his illness, and personal things about other employees, that she should have never shared with anyone. The day came when it was my turn to be interrogated in a private conference room. I was told that I could be fired if I didn't tell them what I knew and so I told them. I told them everything she told me and everything that I had heard. By the end of that week, she was boxing up everything in her office and called me in and really let me have it.

"What the hell did you tell those people?" she almost screamed at me.

"I told them the truth of what I knew, but I didn't go into any detail," I told her.

"What did they ask you?" she asked.

"They asked me if I knew if you were a lesbian, and I told them no, I didn't know that. I told them that you told me that you hired me because you needed a chocolate chip in this cookie too." Which is exactly what she had told me when I was hired.

She rubbed her face and turned red. "I gave you a chance! I told Harold that we should hire you. I told him that you were a country girl who lived on a farm and raised chickens and that we should give you a chance."

"When I came here this place was a mess. It was losing money and the staff was running the show. I worked my ass off to turn this spa around. I came in early and left late. I brought experience to the table, not chickens, and I am far from a farm girl."

"Doesn't matter, I'm suing them anyway. Maybe you did me a favor. They are only using this as an excuse because they know I'm a lesbian. They fired Kevin because he was gay, and so I was next anyway."

By the end of the next week, even the General Manager, Harold was gone as well. I never even got to say goodbye to him. I kept my head down and worked to become a viable competitor in my area. Getting to know my team was a positive thing, and they called me "Captain of the Ship." They looked for me to lead and guide them at a time when I could barely guide myself. This was a new phase in life for me and became my anchor, my passion. I felt important, needed, and was it was my responsibility to guide all of these people to success. This was just the boost I needed for my self-esteem, and I became obsessed with it. It was as though I could feel a part of myself healing. It wasn't my heart, it was deeper than that.

Something was transforming around my heart, something bigger than my personal distress. I had embarked on a new phase in my life. I had awakened a part of me that felt dormant, a drive like I had never known and I felt strong. My behavior was changing in spite of my relationship with Albert. I liked how I was feeling at work. I liked who I was at work. I liked the person I was when I was producing something good, a good that was measurable and recognized by important people. My normal was changing and it began to shift my perception of who I was. What I had written and exercised in my mind for my future vision was becoming manifested and the flow of it was bigger than me. It was taking on a life of its own. I was tuned into the fact that I was becoming my best self so far. The more I concentrated on my career, the more I neglected to pay any attention to Albert and his rages or threats.

I had long stopped paying attention to his comings and goings. I didn't care about his drinking at all once I hired a nanny. Lily was a year old when I hired Consuela. I hired her so that Albert could finally go find a job. We had been here for almost a year and he still couldn't manage to find work. Consuela was working at the hotel as a housekeeper when I first met her. I asked her if she did babysitting, and she said she could if I paid her the same as the hotel paid, which was minimal. I offered her $10 an hour and allowed her to bring her two-year-old son David with her. It was the perfect situation for both of us. She was making more money and could be with her son. She was a motherly type who cooked, did my laundry, hung my shirts so they wouldn't wrinkle, and fed my kids well. I no longer had the worries of a drunk looking after my children, even if and especially because that drunk was their father.

It was the perfect solution, one that I had written in my goals. Consuela gave me daily reports on the milestones that I missed with my daughter. She caught the bus to my home and most days her husband picked her up. Albert was on a constant job hunt, never finding anything solid, but picking up a few handyman jobs here and there. We were still waiting for the house in Michigan to sell and things were getting expensive while I was trying to maintain two households. By the time the house sold, I was already robbing Peter to pay Paul just to stay afloat.

I had written a check from our construction business account that he still held in Michigan in order to keep the electricity on and keep Consuela employed. I knew the account had no money in it, but I thought that some miracle would happen and I could replace the money in time for the check not to bounce twice. I was able to do that for a couple of months before Albert found out and closed his account without telling me. By the time I discovered the account was closed, it was too late. I had written a bad check on a closed bank account and was severely reminded that it was against the law.

The house finally sold and provided me with a very welcome financial relief, but it was still not quite enough to get me out of the financial hole I had dug for myself. Each payday was just enough to pay rent, Consuela, and the past due balances on any utilities before shut off.

I wasn't really worried at this point. I was determined: determined to find a way to pay these bills. Albert was still drinking, but I saw no evidence of drug use, nor did I really care. I almost wished that he was still using so that he could overdose and just die. He was just in the way now. I felt bad for feeling that way. It seemed the only way to be free from his drunken tyranny was to have him leave the world of the living.

I wasn't quite ready to leave him yet, as I couldn't quite meet all of the bills each month and I felt that I needed to at least be able to do that before I took the kids and left to be on my own. Lily was still so young. All I needed was just a little more time. Then I would be ready to leave, never for a moment seeing the reality that I had no reason left to remain in the situation I was in.

So I stayed. I turned all of my focus to my work and the kids. I didn't have the energy or desire to focus on my marriage. I didn't want to, it was over, and there was no fixing it. There was no fixing him and he wasn't about to change. I had learned to live with this, almost as if it was a back pain that wouldn't go away. You just live with the nagging pain of its existence.

I had received my annual review and a nice bonus when my one-year anniversary had come around. I felt great, I felt accomplished and worthwhile - at work. It felt good just to be there. I hated being at home and couldn't wait to get up and go to work until one day something changed.

It seemed as if suddenly I became anxious and paranoid about the people I worked with. I felt myself withdrawing. I was beginning to feel the sense that something was wrong, but I couldn't put my finger on it. While I was at work, planning for a successful future, I had no idea that Albert was at home, planning for the destruction of it.

M. Rene Harris

CHAPTER NINE

A Wounded Soul

"There are wounds that never show on the body that are deeper and more hurtful than anything that bleeds." ~ *Laurell K. Hamilton*

The anxiety was becoming more prominent within me. I felt nervous all the time, but I tried to mask it at work. The bonus money had come and gone as I caught up on bills and the holidays rolled around. Something was missing, I didn't know what that something was and had no way to help myself identify it until I heard it.

I was sleeping, and it had to be about two in the morning. We had all gone to bed, me and the kids. I don't remember Albert being at home, or even when he came home and got into bed, I just remember being awakened by his voice.

As I lay there sleeping, I heard him whispering softly in my ear. I opened my eyes a bit just to confirm that I was awake, but I did not move. I closed my eyes again, laid very still, and purposely continued to breathe deeply and heavily as if I were asleep. He continued whispering softly, his mouth close to my ear.

Quietly, rhythmically, installing subliminal messages into my subconscious. Messages that would have been – must have been – the reason for the sudden change in my waking life. I listened carefully to the words my husband was whispering to me while he thought I was asleep.

"They hate you at your job," he whispered. "Your work is terrible." He continued with, "They are looking for reasons to fire you," "No one there likes you," "You want to quit," "You are bad at what you do." And it continued from there.

A tear rolled from my closed eyes as he said these words to me. How long had he been doing this? What else had he been saying to me? Why would he say these things to me? I couldn't hear any more coming from him, so I moved a bit and sighed. He quickly rolled to his side of the bed and pretended to be asleep. That bastard! What kind of evil lived inside of this man, I wondered? I would soon find out.

The whispering was just the beginning of the evil that was lurking inside of him. He would become worse, much worse, and he would use my only source of peace - my sleep - to display his power over me. Now armed and knowing that he was trying to manipulate me through my sleep by whispering these messages, I started to notice his actions during my waking state.

The change in me must have been noticeable because he became nicer. Much nicer. He would offer me a cup of tea or a glass of water before I went to bed; I would kindly accept and then dump it in the toilet. When he would finally come to bed, I would get up and move myself to the couch in the living room or bunk with one of the kids for protection. I would lay next to the kids and read bedtime stories long enough to fall asleep in their beds with them until they finally asked me to stop. Perhaps that was his doing as well.

Work was going great again and my attitude was improving. I was more determined than ever to succeed, but sadly the damage had been done on an ethereal level. We had gotten a new General Manager who didn't like me at all. He saw no value in my work or my position and asked me to show him what my responsibilities were by making a list of my job duties daily, weekly, and monthly. I was no longer invited to be a part of any decision-making at an executive level. I was no longer invited to participate in any owner's dinners or functions and my visibility within the leadership of the hotel was shrinking rapidly.

Since I had discovered this thing that was happening to me in my sleep - my sleep was suffering. I could not rest and it showed. It showed in my quality of work, it showed in my appearance, it showed in how I interacted with my employees and everyone else around me. I knew I needed to get a handle on this and soon, but my old companion, depression, was knocking on my door. Again.

I knew that if I let depression in again, my life would regress and I could not allow that. I was so close to being able to be free. I couldn't stop now. I needed to push forward through this. I needed to get past this in order to survive. I was stronger than this and I knew it now. I would make a new plan. I went to bed that night. In my own bed, mainly because he wasn't there and I was exhausted. Earlier in the day, Albert had left his cell phone in the kitchen, and I picked it up and went through the photos. I saw a picture that was taken in the dark. He was holding someone's eye open. I asked him what it was and he said it was the dog's eye, that she had something in her eye and he wanted to get a picture of it so that he could try to figure out what it was. I told him to take her to the vet to get it taken care of. He told me to take her if I was so concerned. I thought that was just stupid. If he was concerned enough to take a picture of it, why not just take her to get it taken care of. And why take a picture in the dark of her eye? Why not call her into the light where you could actually see it? We continued to argue about him not taking the dog to the vet, the fight was beginning to escalate and he left, and I didn't expect him to come back that night. I was actually relieved and was looking forward to a good night's sleep for a change.

Tonight is where the past and the present would collide. It was this defining moment that I first spoke about, and it would force me to see things for what they truly, and painfully, were.

I woke up and with my eyes still closed, I took a deep breath. Without opening my eyes, I lay there for a moment. Still. Not moving. Breathing. It seemed like any ordinary day, but this day would prove to be anything but. I opened my eyes and saw him, just lying there. Sleeping, snoring. I scrunched my face in disgust. I hated him. I never wanted to feel this way but I now feel a disdain for this stranger lying next to me. I wondered what kind of mood he would be in today. We never knew what to expect or the temperament that would dictate our day.

I tried to turn over, to stretch and yawn out my slumber, but as I went to move, a burning pain seared up my spine and jolted me wide awake. As I tried to move into a sitting position at the edge of the bed, the pain became excruciating and radiated down into my thighs. Cramping in my lower back and ass gripping me as I headed towards the bathroom. I had never felt this kind of pain before. I felt a sharp stabbing pain tearing in my rectum. My mind tried to understand and identify what this pain could possibly be and what was going on in my body at the moment. What had he done to me? I searched my mind for answers, but I couldn't comprehend how on Earth he had managed to do what my gut was telling me he had done.

As I sat on the toilet crying from the pain and the hurt of what I feared had happened to me. I closed my eyes and held my breath and with trembling hands, I wiped myself. I hesitantly looked at the toilet paper and confirmed my fears. I was confronted with blood and mucus or semen staring back at me. I suddenly needed to throw up. I pulled the small trash can from the side of the toilet and emptied my stomach of all its contents until there was nothing left. My mind raced for answers, but nothing made sense. How and when could I have been rendered unconscious in the night? He wasn't there when I went to sleep, so did this happen when I was already sleeping?

I felt the immediate need to protect myself, but from what? I wasn't sure. I had no evidence except for the pain in my body and the excretions that were glaring at me, but that was not a confession, that was not undeniable evidence that it was him. I had only my gut feelings to guide me and prompt me to protect myself. I had stopped eating or drinking anything he offered me, so how could this happen? His need to control me had gotten worse and had now introduced a new level of fear from the demon who shared my bed. I was trying to force myself to remember. I remember kissing my children goodnight and climbing into bed. I don't remember him being home when we went to bed; in fact, he was rarely home at all. And if he was, he wasn't sober. Most times we didn't know where he was. That's the last thing I remember before going to sleep that night. No, I don't know how my night ended, not because I was drunk or high, I was not into those things. It had been nearly 20 years since I had gotten drunk. It was important to me to always be in control and aware of what was going on around me at all times.

This I had no control over. No control over my body or what happened to it or by whom. My mind kept frantically searching for another possible answer; I tried to think, but I couldn't. I could hardly comprehend what had happened to me, but in my gut and in my heart, I knew, but in my mind, I still could not accept that my husband had done something bad to me. Had he raped me in the worst way?

I wanted to go to the doctor or call the police, but what evidence did I have? Something inside my head kept telling me that I had no right. There was something subconsciously that kept telling me that he had a right to do whatever he wanted to me – that I belonged to him. That I had no rights to my own body, that nothing would be or could be done and that reporting him would only make thing much worse. What would I tell my children? How would they feel if they found out? How would hearing accusations of their father being a rapist by their own mother affect them? What if anyone else found out? Was the eye he was holding open in the picture mine? Did he take pictures of anything else? Did he video it? Did he share it? What if I was wrong?

I got into the shower and scrubbed my skin so hard, it was raw in places. I couldn't seem to get clean, no matter how many times I scrubbed. I masked the sound of my sobbing by biting my lips so hard that I noticed when I got out of the shower that I had bruised them. I looked for injection marks on my body. Surely he must have injected me with something. There were no wound sites, no raised marks, not even anything that looked like a mosquito bite. How was he able to do this? Maybe I am wrong. I must be.

When I got out of the shower and looked at myself in the mirror I cursed myself, I cursed him, and the tears fell again. "You don't have time to deal with this right now," I told myself. "Get yourself together, girl". I found a bottle of Visine on the bathroom counter and put the drops into my eyes to take away some of the redness, but I knew the swelling from crying would take time. When I returned to the bedroom, he was sitting on the bed staring at me and asked me what was wrong.

I told him that I was in pain, that when I went to the bathroom there was blood and I didn't feel well. He continued to ask me to describe how I felt, where I hurt. I told him that I was going to see a doctor; he told me it wasn't necessary, that maybe I swallowed a peach pit and that sometimes when it comes out it can hurt and make you bleed a little. I reminded him that not only do I not like peaches, but we didn't have any. And why in God's name would anyone purposefully swallow the pit?

As I walked out the door and left him sitting there on the bed, I heard myself say, "I hate you." I didn't know if I had finally said the words out loud this time, and I felt bad for feeling hate. This time, I didn't care. I hated him. I hated everything about him. I hated the fact that I was still there with him. I hated the fact that I had children with him. I hated the fact that I ever met him. I couldn't understand why God would allow this to happen to me. Why would God allow such evil into my life? I hated God. I hated that I even believed.

Later, I was at work, sitting at the computer, just browsing. I couldn't focus. I couldn't concentrate on my work. My mind was in a whirlwind of questions of "Why?" I suppose when you start to ask yourself questions, your mind will search for answers to give you. The answers came flooding. Why? Because! Because you're weak. Because you deserve it. Because you stayed in a relationship you were never meant to be in in the first place. Because you're stupid. Because you're ugly. Because, because, because... I felt the tears rolling down my face. I hated myself in that moment. Hated that I didn't feel like I had the strength to make a change in my own life. Hated feeling like I had no control over my own life or my own body. I wasn't safe in my own home, not even in my sleep. Maybe the Devil did have time for me after all. It seemed I was a target for him. He was hot on my heels and he caught me because I let my guard down. I rested. I should have kept running, but I was so very tired. I let the Devil catch me.

I needed to ask myself better questions.

As I looked around my office, I noticed for the first time how nicely the furniture was arranged. I had not noticed before. How the colors matched, the muted tones and the casual beachy feel. The color of the chairs, the woodwork, and it's detail. I was in a depth of despair like I had never experienced when I heard a man's voice in the lobby. It had rich deep tones and a hearty laugh. Then I heard my receptionist say, "Just one moment, I'll see if she's available."

I quickly pulled the compact mirror from my desk drawer and dried my tears. I looked like shit. I didn't have on any makeup and thank God for that or I would have looked like a raccoon. I dabbed my eyes again with a tissue just before she walked in and let me know that I had a visitor. I didn't remember making any appointments, but I agreed to see him anyway. The way my day was going it was probably another customer wanting to complain directly to me and give me a hard time for something not going right.

"I'll be there in a minute," I told her. I took a few deep breaths, and when I looked up again, I looked into the eyes of an angel. He was tall, with dark features, and spoke with an accent.

"Hi, my name is Ben and I designed this place. I see you've changed a few things." He smiled a warm smile and I forced a smile upon my face. I gave him a tour and showed him the small changes I had made to his original design. The changes were subtle. I had added some vibrant orange color in the lobby and moved around a few chairs. Added a few candles, nothing major. I just "homed" it up a bit.

As we walked through, he told me his reasoning behind his design concept. He spoke softly but warmly. He was very kind and his eyes were warm and friendly. He teased me a bit about changing what he had worked so hard on, and when I went to apologize, he laughed and made me feel immediately at ease.

"I have a few ideas on some other things we can do if you want to change the design more. Maybe we can discuss it over coffee?" he offered.

"I'm sorry, I can't right now. But if you want to send me your ideas, I would be happy to take a look at them." I hated having to say no.

He gave me his business card as I escorted him back to the lobby. I had some more sulking to do, and he was not welcome to my personal pity party.

"Let me know if you change your mind about that coffee," he said as he smiled and walked out the door. I smiled and went back to my office where my depression was waiting for me.

I sat there at my desk, holding his business card. I looked at it and felt a smile come across my face again, so I threw it in the trash. I had work to do. But first, I would call my doctor and make an appointment.

M. Rene Harris

CHAPTER TEN

The Courage in My Purse

"Man cannot discover new oceans unless he has the courage to lose sight of the shore." ~ Andre Gide

I sent my resume to a company near Los Angeles. They were building a spa in an existing hotel. I received a phone call for an interview the very next day. We had arranged to meet in two days. I got up that morning as if I was going to work as usual. I had taken the day off in order to make the drive.

This place would be a challenge. It was a golf resort just east of Los Angeles. While the resort itself was beautiful, the surrounding area was industry and ghetto. As I met with the General Manager and the Director of Marketing, I was inspired by the vision they had of making this place a lost jewel, a hidden destination. They were both equally passionate about the vision of becoming a destination resort, the only missing piece was a spa.

That's where I came in. The General Manager was kind and

exuberant as he toured me around the large resort on a golf cart. There were two PGA golf courses, an equestrian center, tennis courts, walking trails, and an Olympic-sized pool at the swimming center. It all looked promising, and when I left, I thanked them for their time.

By the time I got home, I had all but forgotten about the opportunity that had just presented itself to me that day. Albert was clearly intoxicated, the kids were hungry, and he sent Consuela home early, so the house was a mess. I knew better than to say anything when he had been drinking and clearly ready for a fight. But I couldn't hold it in. So I tried a soft approach at first.

"You know, if I had come home and Consuela was drunk, I would fire her immediately," I said to him. He stood there in the kitchen, balancing himself with one hand on the counter, as I started to prepare dinner, just staring at me. I didn't see the fury in his eyes as I kept talking, not looking at him, as I gathered the vegetables from the refrigerator. "What we don't want to happen is for the kids to get hurt and you are not able to help them or get them the help they may need. What if you pass out? Then what? That's why I hired someone. Someone who I can depend on to take care of the kids," I continued.

Next thing I knew, we were standing face to face, and he was furious, raising his voice at me. The boys were standing in the kitchen by then. It was too late to diffuse the situation. The fire had been fueled and we were nose to nose. The boys were afraid.

"Stop fighting!" John screamed with his hands over his ears.

"I can't help it if you're mom's a bitch," Albert yelled at them. Time froze for an instance. I looked at my sons, I looked at him. I stepped right back into his face and said, "Don't you ever call me a name in front of our kids again."

"What are you gonna do about it. BITCH." He laughed.

Clark stepped in between me and his father. "Don't talk to my mom like that," he said to his dad.

"Oh, you think you're a man now? You wanna get in my face?" Albert replied.

I saw something in his eyes that I had never seen before, and I immediately turned to my son and put my hands on his chest. "Please stop, don't do this, he is still your father. I got this."

The look in my son's eyes is a look I will never forget. A look of helplessness, a look of disgust, not for his dad, but for me. I immediately wanted to suck those words back into my mouth. I regretted them the moment they came out. He couldn't help me. He couldn't save me. I wouldn't let him.

An instant disconnect happened in that moment between me and my son. I felt it. I saw it. A disconnect that would not be recovered anytime soon. My heart sank and I hurt for my son. He wanted to protect me and I couldn't let him. I knew if I hadn't, his father would have beat him like a grown man in order to "teach him a lesson." Did I really protect him by stopping him from protecting me? I felt I had lost him in that moment. I had to find a way to fix that. But not now.

Right now, I had bigger fish to fry. Albert left, I could only hope it would be for good this time. Whenever he got drunk and stormed out of the house, I would fantasize about him getting into a fatal accident. I could see his body, bloody and mangled - and then I would see the possibility of some innocent person getting hurt and I would start to pray for the safety of everyone on the roads who would be around him. Not realizing that in praying for the safety of those around him, that I was praying for his safety as well because he always came back, eventually. I fantasized a knock on the door at 2 a.m., it would be the police telling me that my husband had been in a terrible car accident and that he didn't make it. Or that I would get a phone call from the hospital emergency room, he would be in the ICU on life support. I would get dressed, put on makeup, go up to the hospital and whisper in his ear telling him how much I loathed him before pulling the plug.

I would spend the rest of the night trying to smooth things over with the kids. Clark went to his room, didn't want to talk, but appeased me by telling me he was fine. The other three needed my attention, they needed to know that I was alright. We all slept in my bed together watching a Disney movie. It felt so safe when he wasn't there. I could finally get some rest.

The next few days were uneventful. I had nearly forgotten about the interview I had just a few days earlier until I received a phone call with the job offer. I told them, "Thank you, but no thank you."

I was too busy, in my head, trying to figure out how to get the extra money to file for a divorce. Would I need a lawyer? I called a few and the retainers were way more than I had. I would have to find a way to save an extra two grand, or more, for a decent divorce attorney. I was just barely making my bills as it was.

The next few days felt like I was operating on automatic pilot. I got up, went to work. I had no recollection of what I did at work. I would go home at lunch and question Consuela about whether or not Albert had come home, what time he left, did he say anything, those types of things.

I would go back to work until I could leave without the anxiety of losing my job then I would go home, cook dinner, get the kids ready for bed, read a story to them, and fall asleep with them and the next morning do it all over again. I was in my drone routine at work: sitting in my office just staring at the computer screen, unable to force my mind to pay attention to the task at hand when my receptionist came into the office.

"Two men in black suits are here to see you. They look like FBI or something," she said nervously.

"I'll be right there," I told her, a million thoughts going through my mind.

I couldn't wrap my mind around what this could be. I prayed that my children were alright. I also prayed that if they were FBI, they were there to question me about Albert. God forbid they were there because of the bad checks I had written. Maybe Albert had reported it and filed a report against me. It wouldn't come as a surprise. Could this be it? Is he dead? Please God, let him be dead.

I prepared myself, checked my face in the compact mirror, and carefully placed it back inside my desk. I looked like shit. No makeup, my eyes were dark and sunken. I was a hollow shell of a human being. I forced myself to straighten my posture. I smoothed my blouse and skirt and walked into the lobby and saw the men standing there. Smiling at me.

"You guys scared me." I laughed. "Lori thought you were the FBI coming to get me for something." The two men I had met with for the job interview laughed with me.

"We laughed about it all the way down here, we knew we would shock you," Mark replied with a laugh. "How are you doing?"

"I'm doing well, thank you. What in the world are you guys doing here?" I had to ask.

"We weren't about to take no for an answer," Mark said matter-of-factly.

"This is a beautiful place you got here," Phillip chimed in. "Would you mind giving us a tour?"

"My pleasure," I replied.

As I gave the gentlemen from Los Angeles a tour of the entire resort, we chatted about their vision for The Palms Regency once again. I remembered the excitement that I had felt when meeting with them before.

"We want you to be a part of that vision, what do you say?" Phillip asked.

"I say yes! I'll do it, but I need to give my current employer 30 days' notice." I said.

"We can't wait 30 days," Mark replied.

My mind raced quickly; I didn't want to lose this opportunity, I wanted to use it.

"I can start part-time next week?" I offered.

"Perfect, come to the HR office on Monday and we'll get the paperwork completed." Phillip beamed.

"I guess I'll see you Monday then." I smiled at them both.

"Congratulations, we'll see you on Monday." Mark shook my hand.

"Thank you so much for not giving up on me," I said.

"No, thank you! You'll receive the formal offer letter tomorrow," Phillip told me.

We shook hands, exchanged hugs, and the two men left.

Lori ran into my office after the men had left and almost yelled, "What was that about?"

"Oh nothing, they were just friends paying me a surprise visit," I told her.

"They looked so serious, they scared me the way they asked for you and everything," she said.

"They did that on purpose," I said with a laugh. "Everything is alright, don't worry. I promise."

"Are you sure?" She looked at me with narrowed eyes.

"Yes, I'm positive. Don't worry." I smiled at her.

Over the next 30 days, my routine became both exhausting and exciting. I worked part of the time in Los Angeles while trying to keep up full-time hours in Orange County. I told Albert that I was working late to explain the time it took for me to drive home from L.A. The planning stages were getting closer to execution and now Los Angeles wanted me to transition to full-time. I needed to be available to meet with architects, designers, and the construction team regularly. It was a fair request because of the attractive salary and benefits package that had been offered to me, not to mention the time they took to pursue me. I knew that I was being stretched too thin to continue to pull off working both jobs that were so far away from each other, so I dedicated myself full-time to my new job.

M. Rene Harris

CHAPTER ELEVEN

Seasons of Change

"He who has felt the deepest grief is best able to experience supreme happiness." ~ Alexandre Dumas

I finally told Albert that I got another job and left him to pack up the house while the kids and I stayed at the resort in Los Angeles. We lived at the resort for nearly two months while I tried to save a little money. Living at the resort gave me a sense of abundance I had never experienced in my life before. The kids were having a wonderful time. Ordering room service and driving the golf carts around the golf course at sunset. Enjoying the Sunday brunch where they made friends with the Dim Sum chef, who always set aside a multitude of Dim Sum and sushi for them. Exploring the hotel, swimming in the pool, and being catered to by the hotel staff became adventurous for them. It was the summer vacation of their dreams, and I felt like the "Mother of the Year" award belonged to me.

I felt accomplished, safe and important. Albert started to come up on the weekends, and I started to feel anxiety set in when I knew he was coming. I could feel my body tense up and my patience growing short with everyone around me, even my kids. I knew they wanted to spend time with their dad, and as much as I wanted a happy family. I secretly wanted them to feel as much loathing for him as I did. Something inside me knew it was wrong to tell them what a horrible human being I thought he was. I wanted to tell them all the bad things he had done, but I was doing the right thing by protecting them as much as I could without directly telling them how evil he was. I encouraged them to respect him as their father.

I had spent years trying to hide his faults. I had tirelessly covered up his sins in order to protect my children from the man he was. That was what I thought I was doing, and later it would turn and bite me in the ass. Soon it would be time to move. We had to leave our temporary sanctuary and search for a home. The hotel was going to be in a sold-out status, and they would need every room, including the rooms we were staying in.

East Los Angeles was not a place that I found desirable not even to visit. I wanted to raise my kids in a decent area, the place I saw in my mind when I visualized what my ideal life would be like, so we moved a little more inland to Chino. Not too close but not too far. It seemed perfect. The house we found seemed to fall into our laps, it was big and beautiful. It was the largest I'd lived in so far with 3,200 square feet in a beautiful and quiet neighborhood with just about everything within walking distance.

Albert was ready to move back with us. Ugh! I had all but forgotten about living with him. The kids and I were so happy without him. No arguing, no fighting, no hurt feelings. I was beginning to feel safe without him. My life seemed to feel lighter and my future looked brighter without him in it. It was time to make a permanent life without him in it.

When I met with the homeowners and signed the lease, I

purposefully neglected to add him to it. I had the utilities in my name, the cable, everything was in my name. I was squeezing him out of my life, out of our lives for good. Albert had moved the furniture up to Chino and got the new house situated, as I found the schools, a local doctor and dentist for me and the kids. I didn't feel bad for excluding him, I felt as if it was part of my exit plan. The plan I was creating to rid myself of the prison I had kept myself in for all these years.

We moved into the house and everyone had claimed their space, making it their own. Albert decided he was going to become a truck driver. This was perfect! He would be gone for weeks at a time and the kids and I could live in peace. I loved the idea, but unfortunately, becoming a truck driver would have its expenses. Moving had its expenses as well.

All of the money I had saved from working both jobs, even staying in the hotel for two months, had now been nearly depleted. I couldn't figure out where it had all gone even though I had been funding two houses in California and all of the expenses involved with that. Two car payments, insurance, kids starting school which meant school clothes for four kids along with their school supplies. It was expensive, but living without Albert was well worth it.

Now he was back and things quickly regressed back to where they were before, everything except my tolerance for it. My ability to keep the peace, to protect him and his actions had made a dramatic shift. It was as if something within me was speaking to me. I heard it saying, simply and clearly, enough is enough, and we've suffered enough. It's time to do things differently.

I can't explain with any definitive certainty the shift that took place inside of me, but I can tell you this: any feelings that I had toward Albert were now gone. Like a puff of smoke, it was just all gone. I felt no love, no hate, no sadness, no frustration, no emotion whatsoever. I felt nothing. Nothing at all. The interesting thing about that turn of events was when my emotional state changed, his seemed to change as well.

He seemed to discover, for the first time maybe, that I was not the bad guy. He wanted to talk more, express his "feelings." He began running baths for me and taking the kids out to do things. I can only assume he felt the shift in attention as I had gone from paying attention to his behavior and responding; whether his actions were good or bad, it invoked a response from me. Now there was nothing left for him and no fight left in me.

However, he was still desperately seeking it. Desperate at attempting to gain back the control and fear he had over me. When one thing didn't work, he would try another, but he could never hide his true self. A cruel word would always leak out, followed by the immediate apology to correct it, but it didn't matter and I showed no emotion to either the cruelty or the niceness he displayed. He knew it was over, and his actions would become more desperate. The problem was that I couldn't see the depths of his private thoughts, which I had severely underestimated.

If defiling me in my sleep wasn't bad enough, defiling me while I was awake was the next logical course of action. However, I was too far into my mission, into my own plans for my own protection, and save my own life. I had greatly underestimated the level of hatred this man held in his heart for me. I felt an even stronger determination to make the changes that I needed to see happen. But it seemed the more determined I was to rescue myself, the more my outer circumstances became a struggle.

The holidays had come and there was going to be a manager's Christmas party at Phillip's house. I was urged to bring my husband, but no children were allowed to attend. There would be a White Elephant gift exchange, and I was excited but afraid at the same time. Afraid that Albert's behavior would be something that was unacceptable and embarrassing to me in front of my coworkers.

By the time we arrived, most of the executives were already nice and buzzed. Phillip's wife was a nice lady, a very gracious host, and after introducing Albert, I went straight to the kitchen to see if there was anything I could help with. The men gathered in the living room drinking, laughing, and talking very loudly. Albert didn't stay in the living room with the men, he came to the kitchen and stayed right by my side the entire evening. Grumbling about this and that until Dan, the resort Golf Pro, got so drunk that he and Phillip started wrestling on the floor.

Most laughed at the display of drunken ego and boy-like behavior, but Albert was furious and ready to go. The entire way home, Albert made accusations about me liking the behavior, about the unprofessionalism of the leaders of which I was a part, and about me sleeping with all of them. How disrespectful it was for them to behave like that. It went on and on for the entire 30-minute drive home. I had vowed to myself in that moment, as I listened to the never-ending rant, to never take him to another company event.

The General Manager, Phillip, who had been so strongly motivated by the vision of creating a dynamic destination resort out of this lost paradise, had left for greener pastures. We were all so very sad to see him go.

In a few short weeks after Marks' departure, in walks Helen Kim, a South Korean version of a Channel Executive. She was a petite, beautiful, well-dressed woman, who was now our new boss. Helen always wore a layer of pearls around her neck, always in full make-up, and her hair was never out of place. But, she was a pit bull version of a human being. She was as mean and intimidating as she was beautiful. Helen's description of taking on and completing a project was described in her own words as just that. "Get it in your teeth and don't let go until it is complete, hold onto it, shake it like a pit bull." This would then become her nickname among the employees who now suffered under her tyrannous type of management. I was busy preparing my team for the opening of the new spa that we were completion while doing my best to avoid her.

There were only weeks until the construction would be finished, and we were unpacking boxes and placing items on the shelves in our nearly completed space, when Helen walked through the glass doors directly towards me with a ruler in her hand. *"What does she want now?"* I wondered, and as she got closer she held out the ruler, one slightly larger than one you would find in an elementary school child's desk, and inches away from my face, she placed the ruler against my ear.

"Your earrings are too long!" she grunted. "They can only be one-inch-long and no bigger than a quarter."

"Of course, my apologies, Helen." And I removed my earrings and stuffed them in my pocket. There was no reason to argue about earrings.

On Wednesday of that same week, I had a lunch appointment with two doctors who had opened a medical wellness clinic less than a mile away from the hotel. I greeted them in the lobby and led them down the escalator to the restaurant that was located next to the spa. We enjoyed a light lunch as Dr. Lee described his vision of the Wellness Clinic sharing the opportunity with the hotel to bring a higher level of service to the clients that were seeking wellness alternatives. I listened and agreed on most of his points. I saw the potential of a profitable partnership and understood the value of what such a partnership could bring to the hotel without risk.

The server came and with a smile removed our finished plates of salad and asked if there would be anything else. Right behind her, Helen Lim appeared. She appeared like an apparition out a ghost story and sat down uninvited at our table. Trying to hide my shock at the fact that first she appeared out of nowhere and secondly that she had the audacity to invite herself to just sit down.

"Who are you?" she said to Dr. Lee and his companion, not asking but demanding to know who they were. I smiled and welcomed her, introducing her to the two gentlemen in my company.

"What are you doing here?" she again demanded, not asked. Dr. Lee was gracious enough to explain who he was and what he was proposing. "Then why are you talking to her?" again she demanded; referring to me but not looking directly at me.

I was embarrassed and felt ashamed. I could feel myself shrinking right where I sat. Shrinking so low and so small I felt as if I could almost disappear. I wanted to disappear. I wanted to shove a fork in her throat. She smirked, never smiled and then dismissed herself as swiftly as she appeared.

After Helen left the restaurant, I apologized profusely to Dr. Lee and his colleague for the rude interruption.

"Don't worry about it, I deal with her kind all the time," he replied. We shared a laugh and I offered a tour of the spa describing its soon-to-be-public features and benefits.

As we concluded the meeting, we stepped onto the escalator and headed back up to the lobby of the hotel. As we rode up the slow moving stairs, discussing our next meeting at the clinic, there was Helen. Waiting. At the top of the escalator. With her ruler.

We could barely step off the escalator and let the people off who were coming up behind us. When we got to the top, Helen was standing so close that I had to push past her a bit in order to step onto the landing and safely make room for the people behind me. "Excuse us, we almost fell backward," I said with a fake light laugh. We stood there at the top of the landing with her to say our goodbyes as she was not letting me move toward the exit doors with them. Without speaking, she grabbed the top button of my shirt and moved it down with one finger and placed the ruler on my chest, measuring something, I'm not quite sure.

"You need to button one more button on your shirt." With that, she smacked me on my rear end and said, "I'll spank your butt for that." And walked away. I closed my eyes in disbelief only opening them to find her gone. Thank God.

"I am so sorry, Dr. Lee." I was horrified. "I'll see you next week," I said with a gracious smile, as he and his companion left the building.

I marched myself straight to the Human Resources office to tell them what had just happened to me. I was met with a laugh and a *"Don't take it seriously, Pitbull is harmless."* I felt sick to my stomach. Had she done this to other people? Was it just me? I don't even know this broad!

Besides that, I am not a large woman, nor am I well-endowed in that area let alone showing any "inches" of cleavage. That would be my entire chest! I went back to my office and tried to concentrate on what had to be done next. My focus was lost, so instead, I fired up my computer and started looking for another job.

On my way home, while driving, my phone started ringing. It was in my purse on the floor by the passenger seat so instead of trying to drive with one hand and grab it with the other, I let it go to my voicemail. My phone buzzed, letting me know that I had a message. When I exited the freeway, I reached for my phone to check it. It was my sister. She had left a simple message to call her as soon as I got her message. I didn't call her back right away. I couldn't, I needed to think and clear my head before I got home.

When I got home, I was greeted at the door by Albert and the boys. I felt nothing unusual although being greeted at the door was very unusual. My mind was consumed by the injustice and humiliation that I had experienced throughout my day. Albert stood there looking at me, and as I sat my purse on the table he informed me that my father had died.

CHAPTER TWELVE

The Adult Orphan

"To live in the hearts we leave behind is not to die." ~Thomas Campbell

I could not understand the words at first. My father died? Like in dead, died? It wasn't registering.

I had just spoken with him over the weekend and asked him to come and visit for his birthday. How could he be dead? Then it hit me. Like a ton of cement had covered my soul. I was frozen and confused. God had taken my mother, then had come back for my father. It was the emptiest feeling I had ever felt.

As I stood there and looked at my soulless husband and my beautiful children, I felt alone in the world at that moment. I felt as if the last connection I had to life itself was taken from me. I had never smoked in front of my children before; I was a closet smoker, hiding out on the back patio to steal a breath of nicotine when they were out front playing with their friends or sleeping. But now, I had no regard for who saw me. I grabbed the pack of

Virginia Slims from the glove compartment in my car and sat on the front porch with my knees to my chest and let the tears fall as I tried to recall our last words to each other just days ago.

I remembered telling him that I would pay for his airline ticket and that I wanted him to come for a weekend, alone, not with his new wife. I would call down his cousin from Santa Barbara and show him around. He kept saying that he couldn't come but that he wanted to. His new wife would never allow that. She was a younger woman, younger than our youngest sister, and had two very young children of her own. I never got to know her, never spoke with her, unless it was to ask to speak to my father if she happened to answer the phone when I called.

I could feel my heart sobbing. I was grief stricken, even more than when my mother had passed. Perhaps it was because I was there when my mother died. Her transition from this life was expected, and she was in my arms when God came and took her from me. But my father? I thought I had time. I thought I would see him again. I thought I had time, but time ran out on me.

I had often thought that a girl marries a man just like her father, but in my case, nothing could be further from the truth. My father was a provider. He worked hard and served both in the Air Force and the Army. He was twice retired and he still kept working.

In my eyes, my father was a hero. When we are young, we don't know what passive-aggressive looks like. As little girls, we don't know that daddy works a lot because he doesn't want to come home. I saw my father's pain and my mother's anger and was the recipient of both.

As children, I think we look to one parent to lean on for protection, for help. One thing was for certain: my parents were a team, a team like good cop/bad cop, but they were a team. Which meant I had nowhere safe to hide the pain of my mother's abuse. As my father would tend to disagree with my mother over her treatment of me, of her locking me in my room, locking the bars on the windows. I could still overhear them arguing. My father became my hero and I was sent away to live with my oldest sister for the first time at twelve years old.

Memories of my father flooded my mind and I wondered if there was a point, a moment in which he knew he was dying, that maybe he thought about me. Maybe he whispered an "I'm sorry" or a "Goodbye, baby girl" before his spirit left his body. I remembered how he taught me to make his different variations of gumbo, and it brought a smile to my tear-stained face. I remembered how he told me, "There are no men like me left in this world." One of the conversations he had with me at a young age that I didn't understand but never forgot.

I felt unprotected in this world. Now that my father was gone from me, there really was no one to protect me. As I sat there on the front porch crying and smoking my cigarettes, my son came and sat beside me, not knowing how to comfort me, and told me that he was still here, that I didn't need to be sad. I withdrew even further into myself.

Alone and unprotected, I felt even less prepared to face the days ahead of me and what they would bring. I had no money to get home to his funeral, let alone try to get my children there. So I published a poem on Facebook in his honor and signed it "Daddy's Little Girl."

The responses and condolences that I received were overwhelming. And from that dedication, I received round-trip airline tickets for me and my four children so that we could attend his funeral. It was in that moment that I realized that I was not alone in this world. That I had a support system that was wider and farther reaching than I could see. That God could bring into my life what I needed when I needed it. And that I would not need to know where it would come from, but what I needed to believe was that it would come.

I gained a sort of confidence and faith in humanity that I had lost. The children and I packed up to go to Georgia to attend my father's funeral, and Albert was annoyed that I had not arranged for him to fly out with us. To be honest, his going with us or how he would get there had never crossed my mind. But I took the money that had been donated by my coworkers and purchased a ticket for him to fly there separately and meet us later on the day we were expected to arrive. So with a baby in my arms and three young boys, I made the trip back home to be with my family.

My father was given a military funeral but was buried at a different cemetery than where he had already reserved a plot next to my mother. His new wife didn't want him buried next to her, and fighting about it seemed uncivilized. This woman and her children had completely taken over my father's life. She had even refused to release old family pictures to us. My mother's things that were left in the home she insisted on keeping.

Since my father's death was rather sudden, we were, or I was, certain that this woman had something to do with his death. If they would just perform an autopsy, I was sure that they would find some wrongdoing. A wrongful death in some way. But they did not do an autopsy and pronounced a death of "natural causes" due to his age. My sisters and I tried for a little while to right the injustice but gave up as life was waiting for us when we all returned home, but we were still not convinced. No one just dies for no reason. Especially daddies.

Life has shown me that it happens regardless and that it will continue with or without you. Life goes on, in its own time. In its own manner, and no matter how we feel about it, even if we stop, it must go on. So I decided that if life was going to keep moving and not wait for me, I needed to move on with it so that I would not be left stuck where I am. I started saving for my divorce and doing my research on lawyers, and I finally began to move my life forward.

I realized that I had been making excuses out of fear even though I could not identify exactly what I was afraid of. My fear had transformed into some type of energy that was pushing me forward. The fear and the pain had begun to fuel me to not want the life I was living anymore. It fueled me towards what I wanted, which is peace, security, and safety. I was tired of hiding and trying to protect myself. I grew weary of walking on eggshells and wondering what each day would bring. I could no longer wait for the next evil that would befall me simply because I was too afraid to take action. It was time to acknowledge my fear, embrace it and move forward taking it with me if I have to.

M. Rene Harris

CHAPTER THIRTEEN

Out of the Mouths of Babes

"Those who expect to reap the blessings of freedom, must, like men, undergo the fatigues of supporting it." ~ *Thomas Paine*

It was a Saturday morning and I was in the kitchen washing the dishes when Lily, now 4 years old, walked up beside me and began a conversation that would help me realize that I had made the right decision.

"Mommy, what you doin'?" she asked in her tiny voice.

"Just washing dishes, what are you doing?" I replied.

"I want to go to the park with you, can we go see the turtles?"

"As soon as I finish washing the dishes, we can get dressed and go, okay?"

"Make John wash the dishes and we can go now," she told me.

"John is still sleeping," I reminded her.

"That son of a black bitch never does anything you tell him," she stated.

I was shocked. I dropped the washcloth that was in my hands and bent down to my young daughter. I felt the tears welling up in my eyes.

"What did you say, honey?" I asked quietly.

"I said tell John to wash the dishes so we can go now," she said.

"No honey, what did you call him?'

Timidly, she repeated the words. "Son of a black bitch."

"Honey, we don't say words like that. That was not a nice thing to say, so don't say that anymore, okay?" I told her.

"Okay, mom," she said.

She walked away, and I stood at the sink and cried at the evidence that while she was with her dad, she was hearing things that were detrimental to her. Things that were horrible for any child to hear. I shook from anger that she had heard that come out of her father's mouth. I didn't have to ask her where she heard it. I knew. I just didn't know what else he could possibly be saying if he felt it was alright to say things like that in front of her.

I went upstairs, showered and got dressed, as I collected myself and dried my tears. Then I took my daughter to the park. We played on the cement turtle statues that lined the pathway to the small playground in the housing community of homes we now lived in.

I was beyond finished with him. And he felt it. Although he was acting nice when I was home, he was still a bully in my absence. He began doing things like running me a bath and bringing me coffee in the morning. He prepared dinner in the evenings but now had the children wait until I got home so that we could all eat together. He would clean the house before I got home and the video gaming he was doing had all but stopped when I was around. He would even take the kids out for a few hours so that I could have a few minutes of quiet time alone. But his true intentions showed as he continued to demean me to our children when I wasn't around.

I was planning to attend an industry event in Los Angeles in a couple of weeks. A work colleague was planning to attend as well, so we decided we would find each other there. This colleague was the designer with the kind eyes who I had met a couple of years ago. It would be nice to see him again; he was a nice person and very friendly, in a professional way, and I had never forgotten that he had invited me for coffee once. I still wish I wasn't being a basket case that day and had taken him up on his offer.

When I told Albert that I was going out to an event that evening, he got upset and told me I never invited him to those things. I reminded him that he doesn't like those kinds of things, but I didn't tell him that I couldn't stomach the thought of going out with him anyway. I dressed conservatively but made sure my hair and makeup were on point and headed out to L.A.

By the time I had arrived and valeted my car, he was there, texting me asking how far I was. Not Albert, but the kind-eyed man. I texted him back letting him know I was just entering the building. He appeared at the entrance and greeted me kindly with a kiss on the cheek. We chit-chatted as we walked around the beautiful hotel looking at the decor and displays placed for the event.

He was the perfect gentleman and stayed by my side the entire evening. I did not anticipate that, nor did I expect what I was feeling emotionally. It felt wrong because I was married, even though I was married to a bad man. I realized that maybe, just maybe, all men weren't bad. We sat next to each other for the evening's presentation, and he removed his jacket and wrapped it around my shoulders because I was cold. He offered to ask someone to bring me a blanket. I declined because I wanted to feel the warmth of his large jacket around me. I would have crawled inside of it if I could. Then, the party was over, and everyone was leaving.

I was getting anxious to get home to my kids. Ben walked me to the valet to wait for our cars to be brought up and mine arrived first. As we said goodbye, I reached up on my tiptoes to kiss him goodbye on the cheek when he suddenly turned and caught my lips with his. We both looked shocked, then I smiled and said goodbye. I got in my car and smiled the biggest smile I had felt on my face in years. I had kissed a man! I couldn't believe it. I was married and I kissed another man. Even though it was a peck on the lips, I felt guilty and a little dirty because I liked it.

When I got home, I undressed and got in bed and a text message caused my phone to buzz. He wanted to know that I made it home safely. He thanked me for a lovely evening and wished me a goodnight. I could not stop smiling and I smiled myself to sleep feeling as if the world was a little brighter. There was something powerful in the feeling of being desired by an attractive man.

I had never felt this before. But I did know that I could not allow myself to even contemplate the possibility of continuing to feel this while I was married. I prayed for courage to take the steps that I needed to in order to move on.

In the morning, I sat on the patio watching the sunrise. I was having my coffee and writing in my journal and asking for guidance. A sign of some kind. I needed strength. I needed courage. I needed God to show me not only what to do but how to do what I needed to do. I couldn't tell you exactly what I was looking for, but I think I was still afraid somewhere deep down.

I didn't want to allow myself to believe the things that Albert had said to me over the years, but they played like a recording in my mind day after day. That nobody wanted me. That there was no Prince Charming out there for me. That I did not deserve respect. That I was no delicate flower. That God did not hear my prayers. That God didn't care. These words hung around my neck like chains binding me. They made me feel frozen and stagnant. I felt hopeless. In that moment felt worthless. Unwanted and ugly. How could any man be attracted to me?

As the sun rose and the darkness faded away, my phone rang. It was my sister and she was in distress. She asked if her kids could come and stay with us for a while until she could get on her feet. She needed to move out of her apartment and get a second job in order to get enough money to get a new place. She would stay with a friend until she could make it happen but there was no room for her and her 3 kids. "Of course, they can," I replied. I didn't hesitate to help her, and the additional company would be a nice break for my kids.

The kids arrived at the end of the week. It was great to see how they had grown. They had been there less than a week when all kids called me to one of the boy's bedrooms and performed an intervention of sorts on me. ME! A marriage intervention. My boys and my niece and nephew urged me to divorce. I was shocked and stunned, but I stood calmly and answered all of their questions as best I could. I knew it was driven by love for me, but I also knew that they, as teenagers, didn't understand. It was my daughter who came to me and once again spoke her tiny words of wisdom.

"Mom, I want you to get divorced by Daddy," she told me.

"Why do you say that, honey?"

"Because he's mean to you" was her response.

And with that, she was off playing with her dolls as I stood there with a look of shock on my face. I had forgotten that I had asked for a sign and I knew that this was a sign that I could not ignore. For years, I had tried to protect my kids from all of this turmoil, but now it was apparent that I had made them unwilling participants. I had not protected them; I had put my children in harm's way.

They pitied me, felt bad for me, and wanted to protect me. I don't know what they were seeing or hearing when I wasn't around, but it must have been devastating to them. If he was attempting to secure their loyalty to him by bashing me while I was not present, he had failed miserably.

I knew I didn't want my boys to grow up to treat women the way their father treated me, but I had not considered that my daughter could possibly be the recipient of this kind of behavior by the man she chose because I stayed. I was showing her that this was how women were supposed to be treated. By allowing this to continue, in essence, I was saying that it is okay to be treated this way. I had to do it for them; I had waited all of these years and had not done it for myself. I must do it for my kids.

The evidence I needed that it was time to leave and the force at which it was coming at me made me know beyond a doubt that the time had come. The dysfunction and pain from it had gone beyond me and was now visibly affecting my children. I had no idea that my living with this type of abuse had an energy. An energy that permeated far beyond me. It had filled my home. It pained me to know that, even though I had tried to protect my children from this, I had actually made them victims of the same abuse by proxy.

I had no idea that throughout the years, everything that I had endured, my children felt even if they didn't see it. They felt the energy of it and they didn't have the tools to handle this. My babies had been thrust into this life of dysfunction without asking for it. The vibration of the energy of hate, anger, fear and depression had inevitably become my family's core values. These kinds of vibrations permeate beyond the self and into everyone and everything around me. I had no idea that the happiness that we experienced when he wasn't around was because there was no fear, anger or hatred coming from me. I felt happy and safe when happiness was the energy that flowed from me and I saw a clear difference in my children.

It was me who allowed this energy to stay. By not separating from the negative, I had embraced it and handed it to my children as if it was some kind of warped gift. I was telling them and showing them, subliminally, that this behavior, these feelings, were normal. Anger, fear, and hatred had become a part of us. The greatest suffering as a mother who wanted the best for her children; was teaching them that being a victim was the higher road. The time had come to turn this around. I now had the opportunity to teach my children, and myself, that I no longer had to possess a victim mentality. I could be an advocate for my own change. I could be a different example to them now. I could be the fighter for right instead of the victim of wrong.

It no longer mattered that I thought I had done right for my children. It didn't matter if I had bought the most expensive things or fed them the most nutritious food. Those were wonderful things to do for my children. I would have nurtured them to death and done all sorts of great things for them. By teaching them to be victims in the process of all this nurturing was bordering on the same mental abuse I was trying to protect them from.

I didn't realize sooner that this is how children learn to love. They learn how to love by first watching their parents interact with each other. That is how children learn to communicate in relationships when they get older. I was coming to realize that one of the greatest things I can do as a parent is teaching them how you treat someone you love.

My kids saw this relationship dynamic, my emotional ups, and downs — and it imprinted on their little brains every time. I learned it somewhere. Now they are learning it from me. So what was the benefit in "staying together for the sake of the kids," I know now that I was basically making huge mistakes. I didn't give or receive love where their father was concerned, so how could I show it to them? I didn't have it inside me. I thought I had been faking the funk in their eyes for many years. I wasn't. They saw through everything, even the things I kept private.

If we don't love each other, and we don't display love for one another, then that is exactly what is it that our children learn about love. How will they treat people as they move forward in this life? My children, all children, deserve to see parents who are in love with each other. I no longer wanted my kids to be the products of a dysfunctional and loveless family in which they saw (and learned) these behaviors.

I could not bear the thought that my daughter would be treated the way I had been treated. I couldn't bear the thought that my sons would treat a woman the way that I had been treated. The way that I had allowed myself to be treated. If children are great mimickers, they are destined to mimic these actions too. If something doesn't change they will treat others the way they see me and Albert treating each other.

I could no longer stay for belief's sake, or fear's sake, or any other sake. Believing that I would be some kind of sinner if I left. I was supposed to ride this out, right? Isn't that what I had promised at the altar? In front of my parents, my family, my friends.

I had become ashamed of staying and afraid of leaving. But it was my children that gave me the courage I needed to want to be happy in this life. I wanted better for them. I wanted better for me even if I didn't believe that deserved it.

As a mom, it was my duty to make things better for them. I needed to overcome my own fears and at least attempt to do whatever it took to make it right.

M. Rene Harris

CHAPTER FOURTEEN

No More Excuses

"Every woman that finally figured out her worth, has picked up her suitcases of pride and boarded a flight to freedom, which landed in the valley of change." ~ Shannon L. Alder

It was payday and lunch time. I looked up "How to file for divorce" and came to a landing page that had all the forms that you fill out for yourself. I filled out the papers, printed them out, and signed them. This was it! It was the moment that I had waited for years to make myself take. I grabbed my keys and my purse and I drove to the county courthouse.

I sat in the parking lot and prayed for the strength to get out of the car. "Just open the door and take one step," I told myself. I took a deep breath and opened the car door. I walked in, and after finding the window of the County Clerk, I signed in and told the lady in the window that I was there to file for divorce.

As I stood there and handed over the forms to the clerk, it wasn't until she told me the cost and I began to write out the check that it hit me. This is really happening. I could not stop the tears from rolling down my face as I put ink to paper. I had failed. I had to accept defeat. I couldn't save my marriage. It was over. I handed over the payment, and the clerk looked at me with apathy. Apparently, she had seen this reaction many times and no longer had any reactions to the pain that was occurring right in front of her eyes. I forced a subtle smile and thanked her for her time and I left.

I walked out to my car feeling lighter, even though I still had tears in my eyes. I sat in my car for a moment and let the feelings sink in. The feelings of wondering whether or not I had tried everything I could. I wondered whether or not I had done my part to make it work. It was too late now. I made the choice and I was moving forward.

I dried my tears and turned the key to start my car only to be met with a ticking sound. I turned the ignition again. My car wouldn't start. My first thought was to call Albert, but the realization of calling my husband to come and rescue me from the courthouse where I had just filed for a divorce from him quickly became a laughing matter. And so I did. I sat there and laughed so hard that I had to pee.

I called my office to see if someone could pick me up and was asked the question, "Don't you have AAA? Every woman should have AAA!" I called AAA and purchased their service over the phone. I waited a while for them to come out and tell me I needed a new battery. The man from AAA was able to help me get a new battery and install it.

I thanked the gentleman, tipped him, and headed back to my office where I could gather my bearings before I went home to break the news to Albert. The weight of what I had just done had not quite hit me. I expected to feel different. Yes, I had cried when I passed the clerk my check. The cost to change my life was less than $400, and while I felt I was struggling to come up with that extra $400 for too many years, I wondered why I hadn't done it sooner. Then I chastised myself for not doing it sooner. It felt like I had simply checked off a box on my to-do list. My focus was completely on myself, my kids and our new life. $400 and a few minutes had changed the rest of my life and now I was free.

On the way home, I rehearsed what the conversation with Albert would sound like.

"Albert, can we talk?"

"Sure, what's up?"

"I've filed for a divorce today."

"Oh, I'm kinda glad you did, one of us needed to. I'll pack my things and go to my mother's. Good luck to you and the kids."

"Thanks, bye."

"Bye."

As short and simple as that sounded in my head, I knew it wasn't the reality of what would take place once I said the words. Maybe it would go something like:

"Albert, I need to talk to you."

"Sure, what's up?"

"Look. We both know that this isn't working and I feel it's time for us both to move on"

"Oh, you do, do you?"

"Yes, I know that you are not happy with me and I think you

know that I am not happy either. I feel it would be best for the children if we were both happy somewhere else. Not together."

"Okay. But what about the kids?"

"Together we can come up with a plan so that you can see them whenever you want."

"Okay, I'm going to go to my mother's for a while and we'll talk soon."

"Okay. - Thank you. Goodbye, Albert."

"Goodbye."

Then he would walk out the door and get struck by lightning.

I laughed a little to myself knowing good and well that I had no idea how he would react to what I was about to drop on him. So that night I said nothing. I watched him. I watched how he interacted with the kids. Yelling at them for every little thing. Making snide comments about everything they did. I paid careful attention to the words he spoke to me. I looked into his eyes and saw nothing but hatred for me. I watched him huff around the house complaining about this and that. I looked at the lawn that he refused to mow. I looked at the damaged walls from the boys rough-housing that he refused to fix. I listened to him complain about me placing my dinner plate on the counter next to the sink and not washing it after dinner. I watched my children's eyes and saw the concern for me when he spoke to me in unkind words. I took care to notice how my body felt when he was around.

The tenseness was deep in my neck and back. My breath was shallow and short as if I was suffocating. My teeth were always clenched so tight my jaw hurt. The next day, I still said nothing, only observed. Maybe I was looking for a light in his darkness.

Looking for any ray of hope. A reason to go back and correct what I had just done, or maybe I was looking for justification. One last justification to validate my choice. Then I thought about all the things he had said and done and I needed no more justification.

Today was going to be the day. When Lily and I returned from the park, Albert had miraculously appeared in the kitchen. I stood at the kitchen island next to him and laid out the papers. Then I told him.

"I filed for a divorce."

"I'm not surprised."

"You will be served within 10 days, and you'll have 30 days to respond."

He snatched the papers off the counter top and went to the family room and sat down and read them without a word. I stood there at the kitchen counter, waiting for his response. He said nothing. He handed me back the papers and began to walk away. Then he stopped. I held my breath as he turned to me and said, "If the boys want to see me, they know where they can find me." And with that, he walked out of the room. I thought to myself "Okay, cool."

We would not speak to each other for days, and over the weekend, I moved into the downstairs bedroom which had been set up as a guest room. The upstairs master bedroom was certainly more comfortable with its walk-in closet and giant bathroom with the garden tub and walk-in shower. I wasn't about to try to share a room or a bed with him any longer. It seemed wrong now. In my mind, this man was no longer my husband.

Later that night, he said he was going out and grabbed my phone from the kitchen counter, stating that he had lost his and began to walk toward the front door. In a panic, I told him no, that he needed to find his own phone and demanded him to give my phone back. I had thought earlier that day to delete most of my messages to Ian, which had turned from friendly to flirty, but I purposefully left some of his messages to me because I knew that Albert would see them. I knew he was snooping. But now the time had come that he would go in and read them, and I didn't want that. I no longer wanted to give him a reason to attack me. I didn't want that to be the reason that he finally let me go. I wanted to be seen as the good person. The one who tried to do things the right way.

He stormed out of the house with my phone, and I stormed after him demanding he give me back my phone.

"Give me my damn phone, Albert!"

"Go back in the house, you ghetto bitch." He yelled as he sped off in his truck.

I went inside, for fear that the neighbors would overhear the argument and possibly call the police. I borrowed my son's phone and called Ben first.

"He stole my phone and he may call you," I told him.

"I'm not worried, we were just flirting. What do you want me to say if he calls?" he asked.

I thought about this question for a minute and replied, "Say the truth."

"I'm sorry you're going through this, honey," he said quietly.

"Don't worry about it, I'm sorry that you're getting ready to get involved in this nonsense," I told him.

"I'm your friend and I'm here for you. You might want to call and have the phone suspended."

"Okay. Thank you, Ian. I'm so sorry."

We hung up, and I called the phone company and reported my phone stolen and had it suspended. They suspended it, but not before he texted just about everyone in my phone with inappropriate messages calling me a whore and a drug user or asking about who my lover was. Many of the contacts in my phone were employees and business associates who did not even bother to respond or comment.

Later in the night, when he returned, he confronted me for having suspended my phone and commending me for deleting my message replies to Ian. The argument was mostly one way, from him to me. And it felt like it lasted for hours on end. It finally ended when I was able to walk away after he had expended his angry energy. I knew better than to fuel that energy, I felt it was safer at the moment not to. I went to my room where my daughter was sleeping and locked the door. I don't remember when I fell asleep, but I do remember that I didn't cry that night. I didn't feel anything except the need to escape this hell that I had created for myself.

M. Rene Harris

Flies in My Coffee

CHAPTER FIFTEEN

Sucker Punched in the Solar Plexus

"Never underestimate the depths the evil, for evil is as deep as the depths of hell itself." ~ *M. Rene*

Albert had finally been served the divorce papers. It wasn't until Wednesday of the next week when I received a phone call in my office at nearly 6 p.m. that I found out that he had gotten a lawyer. I was demanded to show up in court the next morning at 9 a.m. An emergency Ex-Parte had been filed against me. I had no idea what that was. I had no lawyer, no money for one, and felt as if I had no hope. I sat at my desk and began to cry when a coworker who was leaving for the day walked in. She saw me crying and upset and asked what was wrong, and I told her. She said she knew a lawyer and gave me his number. I called hoping he might still be there. He answered and agreed to meet me at the courthouse in the morning and said I could give him a partial down payment for his retainer before we went in the courtroom.

I arrived at the San Bernardino Courthouse at 8:00 a.m. to meet

161

with my new lawyer, Peter Baker. I had never had a lawyer before, and in my desperation, I had no time to research or even ask how all of this was supposed to go. Due to the fact that I had to meet with a judge in less than an hour, I had to believe that Mr. Baker was a gift sent from God. After all, he specialized in complicated divorces, he took my call late in the day, he took me as a client, and he was willing to work with me on paying his retainer. This must be a godsend, a miracle. The heavens must surely be on my side.

I paid Mr. Baker $250 just to walk in the courtroom with me. We would agree to meet later in his office to discuss my case and, of course, his payment. He took a moment to explain to me what an Ex-Parte was and asked me why Albert would try to take the kids away from me and flee to his mother's home in Michigan.

When I finally understood what was really happening and why I was there, it felt as if the wind was knocked right out of me. The tears had begun to well up in my already red, swollen and tired eyes again. Mr. Baker quickly instructed me to suck it up. I needed all of the strength that I could muster right now. I needed to be strong and appear confident for this hearing and each hearing after.

When we walked into the courtroom, Albert was sitting on right side of the room with his attorney, Rose Michaels, a Latina with something to prove. She was good at her job and she knew it. As our case was called forward, we both stepped up to the front of the courtroom with our attorneys. He on his side and me on mine. Judge Gloria White would be presiding over our case. As the information unfolded, I discovered why I was really there. According to his report, I was a whore, sleeping with nearly everyone I work with, including my employees; male and female. I was a drug addict. I was a partier and never at home. I didn't feed my kids, they had no food, no clothes, no time with me. I had a surgery called vaginoplasty - I didn't even know what that was. I was mortified.

Peter objected to the Ex-Parte by stating that Albert's attorney did not follow the proper protocol for delivering a court summons and allowing us to prepare. He went on to say that I was not properly served as I had just received a phone call at work yesterday from Ms. Michaels's office being told to show up in court this morning.

Albert and his attorney had not anticipated that I would walk in with an attorney, and it happened to turn their plan upside down. I was praying that the judge didn't believe what was being reported about me, and thank God, she didn't. She dismissed the Ex-Parte and set a hearing for nearly a month later. Walking out of the courtroom, I excused myself to the bathroom in order to get myself together. Once I entered the bathroom, the tears started to flow on their own. I went to the mirror and dried my eyes, leaned on the sink and looked at myself. It looked like I had aged 10 years in one hour. I took a deep breath, straightened up my back, put my purse on my shoulder, and walked out of the bathroom into the hallway only to see Albert standing there waiting for me.

"If you stop all this now, I'll stop."

"Why would you want a wife who's a druggie and a whore, Albert?"

I walked away and met back up with Peter and told him what Albert had just said to me.

"Come on, I'll walk you to your car."

We left the courthouse, and I followed my attorney back to his office to go over a strategy on how to deal with this type of attack and a plan of action to try to resolve the divorce in as amicable a manner as possible. When we arrived at his office, which was nearly a half hour away, I took a seat in the big leather chair in his quaint office and was offered a glass of water.

He went over his retainer and cautioned me to be careful during this divorce. He seemed to recognize that my husband was a man who would go to whatever lengths possible to hurt me and that we would need to be two steps ahead of him in order to come out victorious in the end. He also cautioned me to stay clear of any male friends. To mind my P's and Q's and stay on the straight and narrow during this entire process. "The only other man you should be talking to is me until this is over," he told me. I agreed, but I knew my career in hospitality would make that an unrealistic promise.

When I arrived home, Albert was there. He looked at me with such hatred that I didn't even recognize him. He was a stranger to me. There was nothing about him I knew, nothing about him that I could anticipate, nothing about him I cared to know. He was now less than a stranger. He was a predator, and I was his prey. He sat on the couch with an uncaring, smug smile on his face as if to say "this is only the beginning." I went to my room feeling defeated. The kids came into my room and just hung out with me and watched TV. while lying on my bed. It was their way of soothing me. Their way of caring for me while I licked my wounds.

On Monday morning, I got ready in the small bathroom next to my new bedroom downstairs and felt a bit lighter and freer. I looked at myself in the mirror and smiled a forced smile to myself.

I felt better for taking these final steps and said to myself, "Finally, it's almost over." I couldn't have been more wrong. In fact, it was just beginning.

My work had begun suffering tremendously as my anxiety level went through the roof. What had started to become routine and a chance to an escape for eight hours was no longer an escape. I felt there was no safe place for me anymore. Albert had begun coming to my job to see if my car was there. He began following me to see if I was where I said I would be. He had turned detective for his own sick needs and legal gain. He had begun to search through my things and found my journal.

If he didn't write in it, he would tear the pages from it. When I would re-hide it, he would find it and began the process of destroying it again. There was no freedom from him, not in my home, at work, in sleep or in my mind. I began putting most of my personal belongings in boxes in the trunk of my car and would lock it at night, keep the keys in my purse, and put my purse under my bed.

He somehow found access to my private things again. I moved the boxes to my office and locked them up there. My body began showing the effects of the constant stress; I couldn't eat, I couldn't sleep and I couldn't allow myself to believe that this was all happening to me. I couldn't help but think that it must be me. I must be going crazy. I made a doctor's appointment and started searching for another job. I needed to make a change, and I certainly needed to make more money in order to afford this divorce.

My job search went rather quickly, and I applied for a promising position of Corporate Director with a large popular spa chain that had a few locations in the area. I wouldn't have to move, and I would make more money. The title alone was something I had certainly aspired to. Maybe a change in my health, my diet, and my spiritual exercises would equip me for all of this. Maybe making some drastic changes in myself would make me feel stronger and more confident. Strength and confidence were certainly some qualities I needed right now. I met with my doctor and found that I was possibly starting to go through the "Change." She prescribed some Xanax, Progestin, and testosterone to regulate my hormones and reduce my anxiety. I requested that she prescribe something to help me quit smoking. To my surprise, she advised that I NOT quit smoking at the moment due to the high level of stress I was under with my life situations.

"Your smoking is not the worst way that you can handle your stress right now. I would recommend you wait until you have less stress before you attempt to quit," she recommended.

"I heard about a pill that could help me quit. Can I have that?" I was determined to quit.

"Chantix, yes, we could give that a try. But if you notice any side effects, I want to see you right away. Other than that, let's make an appointment for this time next month."

The pharmacist asked me if I had any questions about my medications. I didn't. I just wanted them, all of them. Subconsciously, I guess I thought that all of this would make things better. Make everything in my life magically *feel* better somehow. Make my pain go away but It didn't. It only made things much worse.

The Xanax did take the edge off, while the testosterone and Progestin set off a series of mood swings that would make a roller coaster ride at Six Flags look like a walk in the park. But the Chantix? The Chantix was the drug from hell and aside from many other side effects it would cause me to lose consciousness. The first time was in Helen's office when I went in to confront her about trying to get rid of me. I spoke what I thought was matter-of-factly, but then my emotions got the better of me as I told her of how I felt frustrated by the fact that the spa I had just opened was suddenly taken over by the owner's daughter.

I told Helen how our new spa owner had come in during business hours and with boxes carried in behind her and wiped the retail product from all of the shelves in order to place her own preferred product on the shelves. I was standing right there while this woman came in and did this while refusing to even speak to me or look at me. Helen seemed to be listening and said nothing as I ranted over this injustice. As I stood up to leave her office, I hit the floor, without warning, Bam! I was down. I guess I had fainted. She didn't call an ambulance but she did ask if I felt I needed one.

"No, I think I'm fine," I told her.

"Well, I think we're going to send you to a doctor anyway, just to make sure that you're alright."

She then had me drive to an assigned clinic where I was tested for drugs and alcohol. As I was driving back from the clinic, or rather drug testing facility, I was turning a corner to head north on the side road when I was suddenly jolted awake by the honking of a car. I had lost consciousness again. While I was driving! I never took the Chantix again.

On Monday morning, I got dressed and went out to my car to head off to work. When I turned the key the car made a horrible sound and wouldn't start. I called AAA for a tow to the Ford dealership nearby. While I waited for AAA to arrive, I called my boss to let him know that I would be late and would arrive after I dropped my car off and got a rental. I accompanied the tow truck driver at the Ford dealership and waited for the technician to assess the problem. He greeted me in the waiting room and asked me to join him in the service area.

"Ma'am, when was the last time you had your car serviced? I've never seen anything like this before," he said.

"The last time I brought it here. I think it was for an oil change and tire rotation." I tried to remember if there was anything else. "Is it the transmission?" I asked trying to sound like I knew what I was talking about, although I knew nothing about cars. I knew enough to act like I knew what I was talking about in order to not be taken advantage of.

"Well, it looks like your transmission is melted. Like I said, I've never seen this before and I will need to call the manufacturer."
"Melted? Is that common? I mean, does that happen?" I was surprised. I'd never heard of anything like this before.

"I can't say. I'll need to call the manufacturer. But your transmission and everything around the housing unit is all melted," he said.

I felt fear strike my entire body as a thought crept into my mind. Like a bolt of electricity went through me.

"What could have caused this to happen?" I asked.

"I don't know, it almost looks like someone poured acid on it," he said, scratching his head. He was clearly perplexed about this and seemed to be talking to himself out loud.

"Should I call the police?" I asked, now visibly shaking. "Can you write that in a report?"

I felt in my gut that if acid had indeed been poured on my transmission that Albert had done it. But I also knew that I was fishing for the worst possible scenario.

"Let me call the manufacturer and make sure there is not a recall or defect that we weren't notified of yet. Please have a seat in the waiting room and I'll come back with an estimate. Do you have a ride if this is going to take a while?"

"No, Sir, I don't."

"Give me a few minutes and let me see what we can do."
I went back to the service area waiting room and watched the little television that they had on the counter. I tried to think of

what to do next. Should I call the police? What would I tell them? Was Albert so angry that he would do such a thing?

When the technician returned, he had a faint smile on his face. He had obviously spoken to a few people and he had some papers in his hand. "Thanks for waiting. We will need to replace your transmission and the housing unit around it. The good news is that your warranty will cover all of it. The parts and labor, which will save you thousands. Can you leave the vehicle with us for a few days until the parts arrive?"

"I don't really have a choice."

"We will provide you with a rental car while we fix 'er up and get you on your way. Follow me."

I followed him back into the service office and signed some papers agreeing for them to replace whatever they needed to replace and signing the agreement for the rental car which was also free.

For the next few days, I wasn't myself. I took the rental car out over the weekend and met some my friends from work at a nearby nightclub for drinks. I figured Albert wouldn't be able to recognize the car or follow me or locate me. It was a basic white sedan and I parked it with other basic white sedans just to ensure that I couldn't be located. I was distraught, confused, and afraid. Although I tried to keep my calm-looking exterior, inside I was a mess. Constantly looking over my shoulder.

I tried to convince myself that no one was following me. That no one was after me. That I was just being paranoid. But I couldn't shake the feeling that I was in danger and the feeling wouldn't go away. Everything within me was fighting to stay calm. My mind was struggling so much so that I felt that I was almost unable to breathe at times. I had to consciously remind myself to take a breath.

That night, I drank and I danced and I flirted and started to make out with a guy from work. I don't know what happened, I flipped and got very angry at him, angry at myself. I felt like shit. I needed something, I wasn't sure what. I needed to feel safe but I couldn't. It was time to go home to my kids. I had nowhere else to go and my kids were there with HIM! My mind searched for something, but I don't know what. I had no clue as to what to do. I was losing my mind.

The following Tuesday, my car was ready. I almost didn't want to pick it up. I didn't want it anymore. I felt safer without it. I convinced myself that I was just being silly and paranoid. Albert was acting as if nothing was wrong, as if things were normal. He showed no concern for the car or for me. He showed no emotion at all, and I chalked it up to the fact that I had recently given him the news of our divorce.

I went home and went into the guest bedroom where I now slept and cried myself to sleep with my daughter in my arms. I don't remember what I dreamed that night or even if I dreamed at all. I don't remember falling asleep, but I remember waking up to the sun shining through the bedroom window. I slipped out from my daughter's body, with her tiny hand wrapped tightly around my neck, and prepared myself for whatever battle was waiting for me.

It was finally time for the next court hearing following the Ex-Parte that Albert had filed against me. I met my lawyer at the courthouse, in the hallway the same way we did the first time we had met. We briefly went over the plan for the hearing and Peter explained to me what this hearing might be like.

The judge would most likely have us go through mediation and call a trial. She may want to talk to the kids. I welcomed that. I knew my kids would tell her all about his drunkenness, the swearing, the belittling, the name calling. I wanted her to talk to the kids because if she did, she would surely give me full custody, and he would have to have supervised visitation or something like that. Just the thought of it made me feel hopeful.

We stepped into the courtroom and went to our respective sides and stood as the judge entered. There were a few cases before our names were called. As the judge called each case forward, the Petitioners and the Defendants stepped up to the front and the Judge would make her ruling. They would leave and the next case would be called. I thought it odd and sad that everyone's private business was displayed in front of all of these strangers with no emotion, and then dismissed until they brought more information forward for the judge to hear, quickly rule on and dismiss.

It felt impersonal. Didn't they know that these were private painful matters between couples, between families? Were they not aware that emotions were involved? Some fear, some hurt, but emotions none the less. Maybe that is why they do it this way in order to minimize the emotion and the long drawn out monologs that could come from an emotional spouse or parent whose life is being disrupted. The hearing was quick. I didn't get the chance to give a dramatic monolog on the portrayal of my dead marriage and point at the monster who stood on the other side of this very courtroom.

Instead, the judge ordered a mediation and ordered us to see a family psychologist to determine custody arrangements. I was then ordered by the judge to also pay Albert's attorney's fees of $2,000. $250 a month until it was paid. If I failed to pay on time every month I would be held responsible for all court costs up front immediately. What the hell just happened here? Albert and his lawyer had petitioned the judge for me to pay all of his attorney's fees since he had no job or prospects of one. His lawyer had him playing the role of the victim in this divorce. He was the stay-at-home dad who loved his children and I was the workaholic wife who was careless and cruel.

The judge seemed to be convinced that he was the victim in this marriage. It would be another month and a half of fact finding, income verification, and deciding who gets to keep what. As the week ended, I was drained and exhausted. Home was not home anymore. It was never home, and I longed for peace.

I longed for a place to lay my head and rest. I was talking to my sister in Chicago one day, in the middle of my own pity party, telling her my sorrows and concerns when she abruptly told me, "Nobody wants to hear this ALL the time."

I realized that she was right. I had no right to impose my negativity on anyone. People had their own lives and burdens, they didn't need me gifting them with mine. I stopped talking about it, to anyone. I stopped talking about what was happening altogether. I talked to no one. I felt I had no one to talk to anymore.

Part of me wanted to be depressed over this, but instead it fueled me to continue to fight, instead of feeling sorry for myself for what I was going through. I went through the weekend gathering paperwork and fighting depression. Trying to spend as much time as I could with my kids, but my mind was not present through any of it.

The next week, I was offered the position with the new company and gave Helen a two-week notice. She wasn't surprised. She didn't show any emotion. I don't think she was even capable of pretending to display any genuine human emotion at all.

I began my orientation in a large office at Corporate headquarters with the CEO. The position was perfect for me. I had four different locations I was to oversee, which would require quite a bit of driving, but that was just fine with me. It was going to be my responsibility to bring consistency in service and standards between the remote properties and the Flagship property. I could do that.

When I left my new office at my new job, I was feeling good. I would need to tell my attorney that I got a new job and report my new income to the courts. This would prove to backfire on me later. I began to create policies and procedures to establish uniformity between properties when my objective was suddenly changed. I was now to focus on one property, in particular, South Beach. It was not the smallest location, but it didn't have many of the benefits that the other locations had.

Finding the location was difficult. Getting to it was difficult. Parking was difficult. And a week later I was told that it was closing down and it would be my job to inform all of the employees that worked there. Nearly 40 people were getting ready to lose their jobs, and it would appear to be all my fault. To the staff there, I was doing this to them and the backlash I received was their anger and frustration directed towards me. Even though I was just doing my job, it was a painful one knowing that these were mothers and father and I was taking away their livelihood without the benefit of giving them time to find alternative income in order to support themselves and their families. I felt terrible.

My next objective was to release all of the supervisors at our Northern location. They would not be replaced nor could they work in other positions. It was decided that the positions would be eliminated. Once again, the backlash was towards me, not at corporate, and I offered no explanation or excuses. I shouldered all the blame. I was sworn at, threatened with karma and my car was keyed. I got hateful messages, and just like South Beach, the swiftness in which this was executed did not give them the opportunity to secure other means of income to support themselves or their families. What a way to start a new job.

Firing people is the worst part of any job, but firing so many people in such a short amount of time was mounting tension on my already delicate and stressed out mental state. These actions, I felt I had to take, only added to the emotional trauma that I was currently enduring and I could feel myself shutting down.

I had a long drive to visit our Northern location. I had a regular route that I would drive, one that would stop at Starbucks for coffee, and I knew all of the exits with clean bathrooms along the way. On this particular day, nothing seemed unusual, unusual for me anyway. I got there and greeted my staff there and went to my office. The office was upstairs in this quaint little spa and the staff was well into their day and working. I would only be there for a few hours before I would need to make the drive to the Corporate offices.

I was driving back, down the I-5, listening to the radio when my car started to wobble a bit. Traffic was moving pretty quickly during the early afternoon drive. I was tired and not really paying much attention so when all four of my tires blew with a loud pop that sounded like a gunshot, I was shocked to complete attention. The cars around me were alert, and with sudden and precise detail that it seemed miraculous. I was able to gain control of the vehicle and safely guide myself to the side of the highway and stop near the guardrail. No one stopped to help and as the cars continued to whiz by me and with my hands shaking, I called AAA. Thank God for AAA.

The responder at AAA asked me if I was in a safe place and I told them that I was on the side of the I-5 and that "no" I was not in a safe place. They urged me to stay in the car and that they would dispatch a tow truck right away. I can't remember how long it took for them to get there, but it felt like a very long time. My knees were shaking and they ached. I wanted to cry, but it felt like I was dried out. Like I had no tears left to cry and I wondered to myself "How did Albert manage to make me blow all four tires?"
When the tow truck finally arrived, they loaded my car onto the bed and I rode in the cab with the driver all the way to the dealership near my home. The tow truck driver tried to make

small talk and start a conversation, but my mind could not comprehend all of his words. I felt as if I was in a terrible bubble unable to hear or speak. I forced myself to adjust and called my boss to let him know what happened. All four tires were replaced with new ones. All four tires had screws embedded in them.

M. Rene Harris

CHAPTER SIXTEEN

Riding the Struggle Bus

"Where there is no struggle, there is no strength." ~ *Oprah Winfrey*

I thought the next few months would consist of Albert drinking incessantly and me attempting to not feel anything. Instead, I didn't see him drink a drop; he was calm, too calm. He was civil and as close to kind as he could get without it being mistaken for sinister. This behavior confused the constant fight or flight mindset that I had developed.

I wondered if his attorney had advised him to act like this, to be civil because of the upcoming interview with the family psychiatrist or if he was contemplating more terrorism. The change in his behavior was so drastic that I couldn't concentrate on anything other than trying to figure out what he was up to. The constant driving for work was quickly taking its toll on me and my body. The constant stop and go on the freeways and the ever-present death grip I had on my steering wheel while driving had my body aching and my knees swollen.

My eyes were puffy and dry from crying myself to sleep at night. I didn't know how I was even crying because it felt like I had no tears left. I needed some kind of an outlet for what I was feeling. There was no one that I thought I could talk to, no one that wanted to hear it anymore which meant, at least in my mind, that I couldn't talk about it at all.

Part of me felt hopeless, like giving up on life completely, but the other part of me - the mother, the nurturer, the fighter – knew I could not give up. The hope this side of me gave, though just a sliver, was enough for me to endure and press on. This sliver of hope, as I focused on it, began to illuminate like a beacon. A lighthouse in the dark fog during the storm. I knew if I just kept my eye, my focus, and my energy on this dim light and headed towards it, that it would guide me to safety. That someday this storm would pass. There was hope, I knew it with every fiber of my being. The fear in me began to fade and as the fear lessened, my hope grew. I was regaining my strength even though I was tired. I felt in my gut that it wasn't time to give up yet. Not yet. If I could just push beyond this, I would catch my second wind and gain some strength.

Albert now wanted to change bedrooms; he would take the downstairs guest room and I could have the master bedroom back. I didn't care and told him as much. My gut told me that he wanted that bedroom because he thought the kids would hang out with him in that bedroom, but that was neither here nor there. So, that weekend we switched rooms.

He took his stuff downstairs and I moved all of my stuff upstairs. I was secretly happy about it because I now had the master bathroom which had the garden tub and the walk-in closet. The larger master bedroom had the California King Serta mattress that I had purchased when we first moved. It had all of the comforts that I had purchased. That weekend, after setting up the bedroom, the kids hung out with me and even slept on the giant bed with me upstairs.

On Monday morning, I had finally had a decent night's sleep. I woke to feel a bit more rested that I had in a long time. I showered and dressed and came downstairs for coffee. Since I was keeping most of my personal belongings locked in my car or my office, I headed out to grab a few things that I needed and when I opened the front door what I saw knocked the breath right out of me.

I looked around and there was paint everywhere, on the driveway, on the front door, on the sidewalk, on the siding – but only on my house. There were pictures of my son in an envelope and a couple of CDs (that were mine) right on front door mat.

When I had stepped out of the house, I stepped on them. I quickly moved my feet and picked them up. I walked out and looked at what happened, with my jaw dropped in confusion and surprise, and as I turned to go back inside of the house, Albert stood in the doorway. He was unmoved by what had happened. I called the police who came out and took a report. Albert insisted it was our oldest son's ex-girlfriend, and due to the letter and the pictures, the police believed it. I wanted to know where she lived and wanted the police to go arrest her or something. They took her name, talked to my son and left. A few days later, the incident occurred again.

As I walked out of the house to get in my car to go to work, I looked around noticing there was paint everywhere again, but this time, it was on and inside of my car too. I must have left my windows down a couple of inches, but the car doors were still locked. Alberts truck was parked right next to my car in the driveway but there was nothing on his truck. I called the police to make another report. A different officer this time. He spoke directly to me and said this was a personal attack from someone very angry. Angry at me.

Again, Albert appeared in the doorway and told the officer what had happened a few days earlier. He monopolized the conversation. I interrupted and told the officer that we had these kinds of paint in our home. I told the officer that I thought my husband did it and explained that we were going through a messy divorce. Albert just laughed and once again explained to the officer that our son had a crazy ex, and she had done this same thing just a few days earlier and that there was a report. He also stated that I was crazy and on medication. The officer left with the girl's information and never returned. I cleaned my car and headed off to work. On my way, I called my attorney to set up a meeting so that I could fill him in on what was happening. We agreed to meet the next afternoon. He ended the conversation by telling me to be very careful.

I drove to Peter's office the next day and sat waiting and preparing myself for what advice he would have for me. I stood as he greeted me in the lobby of his small office and we walked back into his office where he offered me water or coffee. I declined both. I told him the story of both incidences that happened that week and he seemed to listen and jot down a few notes. He told me to be very careful and that at our next court date, which was a few weeks away, he wanted to talk to Albert to get a feel for what we were dealing with.

He then notified me that he would not be available for the next week because he was going on vacation with his fiancé. They needed to get away to plan the wedding. He asked if I was prepared to meet with Dr. Stewart, the family psychiatrist assigned to our case. We went over the questions he might ask and how I was to answer them. Make everything about the kids. Say "our children" a lot. It seemed that I had a habit of saying "my kids," and I needed to show that I was a team player wanting what was best for "our children." I listened and agreed.

The following week, while Peter was away on vacation, we would all pay a visit to Dr. Stewart, but not all at the same time. I don't know who was interviewed first that week, Albert or myself as they were scheduled separately. That didn't matter because I would tell the truth; I was going to tell the doctor everything. No matter what Albert had to say, this man would surely know the truth when he heard it. Plus, he was going to interview the kids and that would definitely blow holes in anything Albert would say.

When it was my day and time to speak to Dr. Stewart, the anxiety I was feeling was indescribable. I knew, I just knew, he would be arrested or at least removed from the home, something. Maybe an investigation by the police for the rape of that girl from the music festival in Michigan would even happen. Someone would find her and help her. Once the truth was out there I would be saved. I felt it.

I arrived at the place where Dr. Stewart's office was located and paid my $310 at the reception window. I was asked to have a seat in a cubicle to fill out a pre-treatment questionnaire prior to seeing the doctor. I took a seat in the first small cubicle, similar to the one you would sit at and take the written portion of the written driver's exam. This looked more like an exam than an informative questionnaire about my parenting views. As I sat down and laid the papers before me, tears started to roll down cheeks and I said a prayer. I prayed for God to help me, to be here with me. "Please God, show me that you are with me." I put my head down and picked up my pencil and there was a sudden jolt. Not just within me, the whole room shook.

Then the vibration of the jolt got stronger and the walls of the partition shook with such force that I stood up. I looked back at the reception desk and the receptionist was then standing on her feet as well. It lasted for what seemed like minutes. It was a 5.5 magnitude earthquake. Right at that moment.

God must be with me. This was definitely my sign. The trembling was over just as quickly as it began. "Welcome to California" was a comment that came from an older lady sitting in the waiting room. I finished my questionnaire with my sliver of hope feeling stronger and a bit brighter, turned in my papers to the receptionist and waited for my turn. Sitting there, in this tiny waiting room, I felt as if justice had finally arrived.

"Good Morning, I'm Chris Stewart." I looked up and there stood an older silver-haired man who had a face that showed that he had heard many sad stories over the years. His face was tight and wrinkled yet he had a gentle smile as he reached out his hand to greet me.

"Good Morning, Dr. Stewart," I said as I shook his hand.

"Won't you follow me?"

I followed him back to his office.

"Are you alright? Did you feel that?"

"Yes Sir, I did, and yes, thank you, I'm fine."

"Please have a seat."

I sat in the chair across from his desk and noticed the bookshelf behind him. There were pictures of what must have been his children throughout their growing years, grandchildren, dogs and a variety of books on psychology along with his varying degrees. At first, I was feeling pretty comfortable and waited for the Q&A to begin so that I could tell the story of the monster who I married. But as the questions came at me and his responses in kind, I felt defensive.

"So your father was an alcoholic, but he was a good provider, how's that?"

"So your mother was abusive?"

"So you stayed?"

"Why didn't you leave a long time ago?"

"Why did you continue to have more children with him?"

Then I realized I was looking down at my hands in my lap and looked up at him. He was reading a magazine. Flipping through the pages of a magazine while he was asking me these questions. He wasn't writing down anything that I had said. My defensiveness and his unwillingness to hear me made me shut down. I answered his questions with yes or no answers from that point. Then he asked me a question that made me know this was all for nothing.

"So, you work for this large company? My wife has always wanted to go there. How can she get in? Isn't it members only?"

What did he want from me? Was this how to get his report to be in my favor? I can't do that, it's wrong and I could lose my job. Should I give his wife free access to the spa with free spa treatments in exchange for him to give me custody of my children? I didn't have the power to give anything away. Maybe I could pay for it out of my own pocket. Was I that desperate? If God is truly with me, then doing the right thing would be best. This must be a test. So I answered him in a way that could possibly turn his favor away from telling the judge that I was the better parent.

"You wife can go to any of the spas, they are open to the public."

With that, the interview was over. I would see Dr. Stewart once more, a few days later when I took the children to be interviewed. He spoke to them separately, except for my youngest, Lily. He would speak to her with her oldest brother present. Then he would speak to them all together to verify their stories.

I would discover what Dr. Stewart had written a week later at the hearing. I met Peter at the courthouse only minutes prior to our appointment time. He was running late. He hadn't yet read the report and had asked for a copy from Albert's attorney because he had just returned from vacation and had the court date postponed another week. Peter and I agreed to meet at his office in a couple of days to discuss Dr. Stewart's report. The next couple of days seemed like a lifetime away.

At work, it was impossible to concentrate knowing that I may have ruined my chances of having sole custody of my children because I refused to be bribed. I was trying not to become discouraged by the behavior of Dr. Stewart, my lawyer, and the court system in general. I couldn't understand why this was taking so long.

I couldn't understand why Albert just wouldn't leave. I knew he didn't want the kids. He didn't want me. He just wanted me to stop the divorce and that was not about to happen.

That following Friday morning, I walked into the courtroom to meet Peter, waiting anxiously to discover what Dr. Stewart had to report. As we sat in the lobby across from the courtroom doors, Peter let me read it.

According to Dr. Stewart, Albert and I had both done a good job of not letting the kids know the real reason for the divorce. According to him, we had both shielded the kids from any arguments or dysfunction. According to this report, we deserved shared custody. The kids did not rat out their father for being an alcoholic. They didn't see him that way. They didn't see him as violent or a threat. They saw me as unhappy but a loving doting mother. They sided with both of us.

While this report should have made me proud of my children, I was angry with them in that moment. I felt betrayed by my own children. Then I remembered that over the years, I had done everything that I could to protect them from seeing his drunken state. I dismissed them to their rooms when there was a conflict. I tried to never argue in front of them. I never told them about the things that he did or said. I never told them about the drugs or other women. I had prayed fervently that God would protect my children from all of it and that was the one thing he did.

Now I was mad at God for doing what I asked because now I needed the kids to know what their father was. The moment that I read this report about what good parents we both were, I felt sick. Peter said that we could dispute the report. Tell the judge that Dr. Stewart didn't listen to me; tell her that he was more concerned with his wife getting free passes into the spa than he was about the welfare of my children. I thought about it but declined. I was too tired to fight another fight. I just wanted it to be over and told him as much.

"This will never be over for him, you know that, right? This man is never going to leave you alone," Peter said to me quietly.

I gave him a confused look. "I just need this to be over."

"I understand."

Peter and I made our way into of the courtroom, and when it was our turn to stand before the judge, both sides agreed to adopt Dr. Stewart's report as is and we were ordered to attend a mediation and return in another month for a child custody hearing.

The next two months were appointment after appointment for the mediation process. There were child care classes in order to teach us how to communicate the divorce to young children.

I made my way to Rose Michaels's office early on a Wednesday morning, the 10th of the month as instructed, to make my first payment. When I walked into the office, I was surprised at how nice the staff was. I had expected them to be mean and ruthless as she was in the courtroom. I had expected them to be short tempered and disgusted with me because of all the things they must have heard about me from Albert. But they were friendly.

I told them I was there to make a payment to the attorney and gave them all of the information. The looks on their faces were shocked as if they could say out loud "Oh, so you are the one!" I knew then that there was no confidentiality in that office. I simply smiled and answered their questions. When they asked where I would like the monthly invoices to go to, I gave them my office address. I told them if they sent them to our home, I would never get it. The receptionist, who was a young man, possibly a paralegal, looked sad for me. I told him to have a good day, handed them the check (praying it wouldn't bounce) and left.

Then, of course, there were the actual meetings with the mediator. As we sat together in her office, Albert had told her that he wasn't staying in the state of California, that he couldn't make a living here and that he wanted to take the two younger children with him and that I could keep the two older children.

She tried to explain to him the dangers that happen in the psyche of children when you separate siblings. She informed Albert that studies show severe psychological trauma happens when siblings are separated. He argued that it was what he felt was best because he was unable to find work as a builder in California due to unions and Mexicans. He informed her that we had property in Florida he would build a house on and felt the building market was much better in Florida than in California. Then the mediator asked the perfect question: "If you move to Florida, how will you ensure the children see each other and their mother?"

"She can pay for them to fly back and forth," he stated.

"Have you thought about the fact that this will cause separation anxiety for your children? Taking children away from their mother has profound effects on children that will last over the span of a lifetime."

"I'll move," I replied. "My mother had sent me to live with my sister when I was young, and it was very painful. Steven doesn't like to fly, he gets airsick, and I think he is too young to supervise Lily on a flight that long. The thought of it scares me. I'll move; without my children, I have nothing to stay here for."
Albert's eyes welled with tears although he was trying to fight it. I looked at him and for the first time in years, I saw compassion. I saw a deep sorrow in his red watery eyes.

"You're not moving! You're going to stay here and be with that guy you're having an affair with!" he yelled.

"Mom? Are you currently having an affair?" asked the mediator with a surprised look on her face.

Albert glared at me as he waited for my answer.

"No, ma'am! And I have no reason to stay here if he is going to move my children away from me. It would be silly and cruel to have the kids fly back and forth across the country like that for no good reason"

As I spoke, the moderator began writing for her report.

"So Mom is going to move so the kids don't have to fly back and forth, Mom doesn't want to cause the children distress by the long-distance custody sharing. Dad is moving to Florida to build a house on the property you already own. Does that sound correct?"

"Yes, that's correct," I agreed. Albert simply nodded. "I will submit my report to the court. Good luck to you both."
I was hopeful that the compassion that I saw in Albert's eyes in

that moment would cause a change in the momentum of his destructive actions towards me. We left, I went to work and he went home.

CHAPTER SEVENTEEN

Common Ground

"Even if all the doors are closed, a secret path will be there for you that no one knows." ~ Dr. Jabir Khalil

I have no idea why I thought anything would be different, but I did. I had to hope. I had to believe that I was doing the right thing by severing this toxic relationship. I had to save my children. I had to save myself. Even though I had hoped for peace in the home we shared, I still kept my most personal belongings, business, legal, and financial papers locked away from Albert.

Lily was too young to understand what was happening around her, and thankfully we both treated her little mind with care and concern, or so I thought. We both tried to do as much with her as we could, like going to the park, going out to play, things like that. But there were days when she wanted both of us to do something or go somewhere with her. She wanted her mom and dad with her, together, at the same time.

On the days she insisted on punishing me this way, I would sit in the back seat with her as he drove. These days rarely ended well. For the most part, we were cordial to each other as we tried to determine who would get what in the divorce. Time was getting closer to the next court date. It was time to finalize the distribution of all of the things we had spent the last 20 years accumulating.

During this time, I would sit out on the patio in the morning, greeting my day with prayer and writing in my journal. I needed to figure out what my next steps would be. I realized that I had a choice as to what I wanted the next part of my life to look like. What would life be like without fighting, without fear, without cleaning up vomit, without walking on eggshells or watching my back all the time? What would it be like to sleep in peace? I could only imagine how good it must feel to be free. Free to think my own thoughts without criticism. Just Free.

One morning Albert came out to the patio with a cup of coffee to join me. We sat there in silence and for a few moments drinking coffee and enjoying the sunrise when he got up to refresh his coffee. He asked me if I would like mine refreshed as well. "Sure, thanks." I never gave a second thought that the gesture might be anything other than a kind gesture since he was going in the kitchen anyway. He came back with both cups of coffee. We sat again and drank our coffee.

"So you're not going to stay here?" he asked.

"Of course not. I have nothing to stay for," I replied.

"Where you gonna go?"

"I'm going to go to Florida since that is where you're going. I can't see the kids flying back and forth by themselves. I can't do that to them."

He looked at me for a few seconds and took a deep breath. With a slight nod of his head as if he had understood what I was saying. The conversation was over and he took his cup of coffee and went back inside. No harsh words, no mean looks, no emotion at all. I continued to write in my journal, sip my coffee and enjoyed the quiet morning. Wondering what my life in Florida would be like. Lily woke up and walked out the patio doors in her pajamas and crawled up into my lap rubbing the sleep out of her eyes.

"Good morning, Sunshine," I said as I lifted her up into the cradle of my lap.

"Morning, Mommy."

"Hungry?"

She nodded her head yes, but we sat there for a few minutes snuggling and basking in the rays of the warm morning sunlight.

I prepared a quick breakfast of a Cheerios in her favorite bowl and the boys soon came down to join her. We decided we were going to take a day trip to the local flea market again. We stayed out past dinner and got home in time to prepare for bed. It was a beautiful day, one without stress and anxiety. It has been quite a while since we've seen a day like that.

On Monday morning and I packed up all of my income statements and bills for Peter. Preparing for the next court case that would decide how everything would be divided. This time, Peter would submit all of the information to the court prior to the next court date for the judge to evaluate. Sometime during the previous evening, my glasses were broken and were placed on the kitchen island for me to find them. Pieces were missing and it was impossible to fix them so I went the next morning to buy a new pair.

I found a pair of sassy Dolce and Gabbana frames with transition lenses. I was so proud of my purchase which ended up being less than a couple hundred bucks. The glasses fit my face nicely and added a little bit of pizazz to my look. I needed that right about now. I had no idea this simple and sparkly pair of knock-offs would become a major part of my story.

Throughout the week, I received many compliments on my new glasses, but I also received comments about my weight. I had lost much of it and so quickly that my clothes didn't fit anymore. People were asking if I was sick, I didn't look well, I didn't look healthy because I had gotten so thin, and my clothes were now two sizes too big. I didn't feel well anymore. I didn't feel healthy, I didn't feel happy, and it was expressing itself through me in every way. I had no appetite and I was subconsciously afraid to eat at home even when I cooked and knew what was in it. I was living on coffee and cigarettes and would grab a bite from time to time while I was on the road. I had become paranoid, thinking Albert was hiding behind every tree and bush. I wasn't sure why I was feeling like that, but I would just get the feeling that everything I did and everywhere I went - he was there, just watching me.

It was time for court again. The judge would have everything she needed to rule on who would get including the kids. She would tell us when Albert would get to visit and how often. I was ready - I was praying and reached out to all of my family and friends and asked them to pray for me as I prepared myself to go into court. I arrived at the San Bernardino County Court House and parked my car in the back parking lot when I saw Albert's truck.

As I sat there in my car, in the parking lot, praying for this ruling, I was able to calm myself - to breathe. I turned off the car, straightened my new suit that fit nicely and with my new glasses on my face; I walked in with my head held high, ready for what the day might bring.

Flies in My Coffee

CHAPTER EIGHTEEN

The Consolation Prize

"When you play the game of life, you may not win the big prize but you always get to choose your parting gift when you leave."
~ M. Rene

Peter was already sitting inside the courtroom, three rows back with the case paperwork spread out on the bench when I walked in and slid into the aisle to join him. There were two cases ahead of us so it gave him a few more minutes to prepare for my particular case, which he was clearly not prepared for. Albert was there, sitting on the other side of the courtroom with Rose Michaels, who was locked and loaded and ready to fire with both barrels.

I watched Peter as he anxiously shuffled through my file, gathering my financial information, sorting and resorting papers, and I looked over and watched Albert and Rose sitting confidently, looking straight ahead. No shuffling of papers, no nothing. Just prepared and ready. A sick feeling fell upon me and

I whispered a silent prayer. My enemy had an army, prepared and ready to fight. I had a broken slingshot and a pebble to defend myself with. My courage dwindled quickly.

Albert took the stand first. He told of how I was never there, how I spent money frivolously, and how we never had food. How I always bought myself new clothes and shoes and never bought anything for the kids. He then mentioned my new glasses and how I had spent several hundreds of dollars on them while the children went without food and shoes or clothes that did not fit. He talked about how he would prepare dinner for the family and set the table and how he and the kids would sit and wait for me to come home so that we could have dinner as a family. He portrayed himself as a house husband who cooked and cleaned while I was out gallivanting until late in the night without caring for my family. As I listened with tears in my eyes, I looked over at Peter who was texting on his phone and not paying attention to what was coming out of this man's mouth.

Then it was my turn. Albert stepped down from the stand and took his seat back over next to Rose Michaels. As I took the stand, I was reminded that I was still sworn in and reminded of the warning if I perjure myself. I wanted to yell that he was a liar and to put him in jail for perjury and defamation of character and being an asshole. There must be a law for being an asshole. I asked Peter what I should do and he simply replied, "Tell the truth".

I sat down, nervous, sad, and angry at Albert's testimony. When asked about the truth of the situations that Albert had stated, I spoke my truth. I was at home on many evenings by unless work or traffic warranted otherwise, which was not that often. Me and the kids went shopping every weekend, I had even bought Clark a pair of Lucky Jeans at a whopping $120 a pair. There was nothing that my kids wanted that I didn't make a way to give them. It wasn't always new - we loved shopping at thrift stores and flea markets. I shopped at the local Whole Foods co-op so that my family could eat healthy and wholesome foods. By the time I got home for dinner, the kids had eaten and I would eat alone, or sometimes if Albert lets them, they would sit at the dinner table with me while I ate. Then Rose Michaels asked about my new clothes. I explained the weight loss and how my clothes were falling off of me and people asking me if I was sick. I explained that the rapid weight loss was due to stress and the baby weight falling off. The judge asked if I was alright, if I was healthy. I answered yes. Then Ms. Rose Michaels asked about my glasses. Confused as to why she would ask about my glasses, I told the court that the glasses were not that expensive, that my glasses had been broken. I could not find all of the pieces to glue them back together or I would have simply fixed them as I had many times before. Ms. Michaels then entered into evidence either the receipt for my glasses which Albert would have had to have taken from my bedroom, or a quote on what my glasses would have cost without insurance. I was not permitted to see the evidence that was presented to the judge. I tried to explain that that was not an accurate receipt when the Judge had the bailiff take my glasses from me and bring them to her. She concluded that the glasses looked expensive and that hers cost $700 and she was sure that mine cost much more. She gave me 48 hours to present the accurate receipt before she ruled.

Over the next two days, I scrambled to find my receipts and insurance information but could not find anything. It was missing. I went to Vision Plus and got a copy of the receipt. I went to the main office and got a copy of my insurance claim and EOB and took them all to Peter's office. I felt good that I was able to gather all of the proof for the courts and trusted that Peter would submit them right away on my behalf. It was not until later the next week as I was in the bathroom getting dressed when Albert walked up to me with paperwork from his attorney stating that I would have to pay him alimony of $600 a month and child support of $1,645 a month until he either dies or remarries. If I could have rubbed a genies lamp and asked for any one thing in the world in that moment. I would ask for some horrific and agonizing disease to enter this man's body.

I couldn't help but think that this phrase must be the reason why so many spouses disappear every year. Lily is 4 years old; I would have another 14 years paying this man to sit on his ass even after the older kids are grown and gone. I felt sick. What kind of justice was this? What happened? How could this be? I called Peter to find out if this was true and his reply was, "Oh yeah, I got that too, I was going to call you and let you know." I was not as distraught as I thought I should be. This time, I was angry. So angry at the world, at God who I felt had betrayed me.

The days seemed to go by at a snail's pace and I was just floating aimlessly through them with no direction. When the 15th of the month came, I wrote two separate checks to Albert and handed them to him in the kitchen. I paid him money to still lived in my house while I still paid all of the bills. Something inside of me sank deeper when I saw the smirk on his face. It felt as if something had died even more in that moment as I looked at the man who stood before me who I had once loved. Was it possible to feel more dead than dead inside? I couldn't feel anything before but suddenly I desperately needed to feel something. Anything. From anyone and it didn't matter who. I was on a mission to feel something and that led to a one-night stand with a man who had been pursuing me for months. I immediately regretted my actions and I felt completely gross inside.

I had never cheated on Albert before, and even though we were legally separated and he was destroying my life and being paid to do it, Albert had been the only man I had been with since I was 18 years old. This man who play video games while torturing my spirit was all I knew. Still, I felt that what I had done was wrong. When I returned home from my afternoon tryst with this other man, I showered for a long time and went to bed. Then the stalking began. Not only from the man who I tried to ignore after sleeping with him but from Albert too. Somehow knew something big was up. I would see Albert's truck in parking lots at various places I went. At first, I thought I was just seeing things. I thought it was my guilt making me paranoid. Then he began calling my HR office and my boss and leaving messages, and soon I was called into the corporate office and was told that my position had been eliminated. It was a kind gesture because they could have simply fired me. Because of his harassment. I was given two months' severance pay and sent on my way.

I left the corporate office and went straight to my attorney's office to tell him that I had been let go. I had no idea what I would do to not only take care of my family, but to also pay the rest of the attorney's fees, child support, and alimony to this vengeful man. I then went to Rose Michaels's office to pay and notified them that I had been terminated and would still do my best to make my payments on time. Ms. Michaels emerged from her office and took my payment in person. She looked sympathetically into my red and swollen eyes and asked me if I was okay. She seemed to be genuinely concerned and that was nice. I shook my head, unable to speak and left.

Peter had submitted an amendment of my financial information in order to modify my income and expense declaration. The judge had set another court date because Albert's response was that I had quit my job so that I wouldn't have to pay him. The following weeks were spent with me at home in bed. I had become too depressed to eat, shower, or dress. The children spent much of their waking time in my room just hanging out with me. When the court date came, I was notified that Albert was now representing himself, his attorney had fired him. Imagine that. She had removed her firm from representing him after my last visit to their office.

The child support and alimony were set at zero; Albert did not fight it and agreed with a nod of his head. The judge ordered that we keep any credit or debt that were currently in our names. Albert would keep the property in Naples and I would keep my 401k which had now been nearly depleted from borrowing against it to finish paying off my attorney.

The judge kept jurisdiction over the case in California even though we had both agreed to move to Florida and we were ordered to never live in the same house again. I couldn't agree more.

Until we established residency, California would be the home of residence for our children. I had no job, nowhere to go, no hope, and no faith. It took a month before Albert and I could talk on partially civil terms. The anger and resentment was so thick in that house that you needed fog lights to see your way from the front door to the back. It was time to discuss the next steps and we both knew it.

It was abnormal for me to wake up on a weekday morning with no job to go to, but here it was, mid-week, and I had no job. I woke up early and made a pot of coffee, went out onto the patio with my journal in hand. As I sat there thinking where to begin, a voice inside of me said, "Begin at the beginning."

Begin at the beginning? What was that supposed to mean? I was in the middle of the deepest darkest hole I could imagine, so where is the beginning, that was silly. Then I heard the voice again. A still, peaceful voice, almost like a thought crossing my mind and it said again, "Begin at the beginning." I closed my eyes and meditated on the statement.

Begin at the beginning.

When I opened my eyes and put my pen to the papers of my journal, the words seem to write themselves.

Today, just because the sun rose in the sky again, is a new day. Today, I can begin again. Each new day is a new beginning.

Where do I want to go from here? As I write the story of the next chapter in my life, how will it begin? I start today, right here, right now. Where do I want to go now? What do I want to do now? I can choose to do anything, be anywhere, and be with anyone. What is it that I want? I had to think about that question for a while.

What is it that I want now? Now that I am no longer stuck. Could I see the blessing in losing my job? Yes, I no longer had to pay this man to live in my house. Could I see the blessing in the rest of all that has happened? Well, that may take some time but I will look for them. I choose to find them.

Then I remembered something. Something that I had read not too long ago. When you see something in someone that irritates you, something you really don't like, it is a mirror reflection of you. So I began to write those things that I was irritated by, to see if I could identify what was wrong inside of me. I needed to see what I needed to change about myself in order to be the kind of person that things like this didn't happen to. Who is the person I want to be now and what do I need to change about myself in order to become the person I want to be? The person I know that I feel I need to be in order to have a peaceful more fulfilled life. Can I find her in this deep dark hole? Is she breathing? Does she have a pulse?

I was still breathing which meant I was still alive. I smiled to myself. I am still alive so life is not done with me. Albert then came outside and sat with down with his coffee. "So what are you going to do, what's the deal?"

"I'm going to live with my sister in Florida," I had decided. "It'll take me about a month to get myself together and find a place for me and the kids."

Albert smirked then said, "We're going to drive from here to Michigan and spend the summer at my mom's. Then we'll drive down to Florida and I'll drop the kids off with you if you've got yourself together. That will give me time to get myself together before it's time for me to have them."

It sounded like a plan. The kids would be on summer vacation, with their grandparents and cousins, aunts, and uncles, and I would have the time to find a job, a place to live, and have everything in order for them to come to their new home.

I looked around in wonder at all the things we had accumulated over the last 21 years. Things that I had bought, things we had decided on together. Things we would now have to sell, give away, or throw away. I had little money left now. Enough to buy a plane ticket to Florida and ship three large boxes.

Albert had made it clear that he would not take anything that belonged to me with him in the trailer he would be pulling. The trailer he had used my relocation money to purchase instead of hiring a moving company when we first moved to California. I didn't care anymore. I only wanted to keep my mother's things. Things like her tables that she had since my childhood, her mink coat that was gifted to me by my father when she died, and a few other things that I could not ship or carry on the plane with me. I pleaded with him and he finally relented and told me to set them aside in the garage and he would pack them and deliver them to me when he and the kids got to Florida. It was a relief and I thanked him.

During my normal morning routine of coffee on the patio on the following morning, Albert woke up and joined me. After a few moments, we decided that we would have an open-house-type garage sale over the weekend and invite our friends over first so that they could buy what they wanted before we opened it up to the public. It sounded like a good idea so I agreed.

I reached out to my landlord and explained my need to break our lease. I told her about the divorce and the move, and she was nowhere near sympathetic to my plight, but she thanked me for giving her a heads up.

"I will be leaving first and my now ex-husband and the kids will be leaving later that week," I told her.

"Just make sure that he leaves the keys and the garage door opener somewhere that I can easily find them."

"We'll leave the house key in the box by the side entrance of the garage and the other keys and garage door opener will be left in a kitchen drawer," I told her.

"Are you sure he will do it? Is he responsible enough to make sure things are taken care of? He's not on the lease so that makes you responsible for making sure the home is left in good condition."

"All I can do is make sure that I leave instructions for him and hope for the best. Here's my cell phone number, please call me if things are not left in an acceptable way." I wrote my cell phone number on the back of an old business card and left it for her.

"Good luck to you and safe travels."

"Thank you, Sasha, best of luck to you as well."

"I'll place an ad in the local paper putting the house up for rent and let you know if someone is interested in seeing it. I may not be able to give you 24 hours' notice if someone wants to see it, can I send them anytime?"

"Anytime, just give me a call and let me know they're coming."

I did my best to organize the mess we were making between packing what we would be taking with us, the things we no longer wanted and the things we would be selling at the open house over the weekend. The kids were not at all excited about the new journey. They had made friends here, good friends. The oldest two had girlfriends and were in love. The kids didn't want to leave California and they certainly didn't want to take a road trip with their father across the country. I felt for them and my heart grieved that I would be without them for the summer while I went to prepare a new life for us.

The next morning, I followed my normal routine of waking up, putting on the coffee, grabbing my new journal and placed myself on the patio to greet my day. I continued to write what I wanted the next part of my life to look like. For the first time in a very long time, I was able to see a brighter future ahead of me. Imagining what life could be like if anything was possible for me, was a new inspiration. I could now see a glimmer of light at the end of my tunnel. I took a deep breath and looked up at the dawn coated sky and released it. I released the finality of it all through one breath. I closed my journal and closed my eyes and whispered a prayer. "Please show me that I'm on the right path."

When I opened my eyes to prepare to write again, Albert came out with a cup of coffee and sat in the chair next to me. I didn't hear him come in from work. We said nothing for a moment. He had begun working the third shift so we rarely crossed paths these days.

"The landlord has put the house in the paper and said if someone wants to see it she'll call me but we may not get a lot of notice." I let him know.

"That's fine," he said, not looking directly at me.

"I told her that you would lock up the house and leave the garage door key in the box next to the side entrance, the other keys, and the garage door opener needs to be left in the kitchen drawer."

"That's fine," he said again without looking at me.

"I found a home for Petri, the parakeet me and the kids bought on one of our weekend trips to the flea market about a year earlier - I'll be dropping him off at Anette's the day before I fly out."

He offered no response.

Shaking my head in exasperation and announced: "I'm going to go get some packing boxes and I'll be back before the kids wake up."

I closed my journal and got up to walk away when he grabbed my hand.

"Are you sure about this?"

"Yeah, I'm sure," I said looking directly into those piercing blue eyes that once caught my attention all those years ago. I saw nothing. I felt nothing. No love, no hate, just nothing. I pulled my hand away and went upstairs to take a shower.

My mind wondered where I could find boxes and what size I would need. I got out of the shower and dressed in jeans and a t-shirt. Standing at the bathroom sink while putting on mascara, I heard a knock at the bedroom door. "Come in," I said. Thinking one of the boys had woke up. It was Albert. "You left your coffee downstairs, I warmed it up for you."

"Thank you," I said, never looking down but looking at him through the mirror wondering why he was being nice to me. He sat the coffee on the counter next to me and left. I had music playing on the radio from the bedroom just loud enough for me to hear the subtle classic rock while I dressed and prepared for my day. Without thought, I grabbed the cup of coffee and put it to my lips to take a sip when I felt something firm touch my lips.

I spit the coffee back in the cup and looked down and saw the surface of the coffee covered in dead flies. I looked at it. I just stood there and looked at all of the dead flies floating in this bright yellow cup. My favorite cup. I spit in the sink and brushed my teeth again, but I could still feel the wings brush against my lips and the firm dead body on my tongue. I spit again and washed my lips with a washcloth. I could still feel it.

I took the cup down to the kitchen where Albert was standing.

"What the hell is this?"

"What?"

"Look at this!" And I put the cup in his face.

"Oh, they must have gotten into it when you left it outside."

I walked away from him, feeling provoked enough to hit him with that cup. I knew that if I so much as pushed him, he would call the police and claim assault. I dumped the coffee and the flies down the sink and threw the cup in the trash. I got in the car and the hot tears began to roll down my face as if on cue. But not out of hurt, I was angry. I drove aimlessly for a while before finally stopping to pick up three large boxes from the local Pack and Send.

When I got back home, Lily was awake, but the boys were still sleeping. I had to quickly gather my emotions and put on my mommy hat.

"Good morning, Sunshine!"

"Good morning, Mommy."

"You're up early, are you hungry?"

"Yup! Mommy, guess what?" she said as she followed me into the kitchen.

"What, baby?"

"Daddy said I could set Petri free, we took the cage outside and opened it and he flew away."

I looked at her in horror.

"Don't be sad, Mommy. Daddy said he would be with his family now and that it was okay."

I could not respond. I just stood there frozen. I had to quickly find a "Good Mommy" response so that she didn't feel as if she had done a bad thing. "I'm sure he will find his family and be very happy now."

She smiled and sat to eat the bowl of cereal I had prepared for her. I went upstairs to start clearing my closet. I couldn't wait to get away from this place, from this man. At this point, I didn't care what stayed and what went, but as I started throwing things into my assembled boxes, I realized that I needed to care what I took. I only had three boxes. I had to begin a new life with three boxes of whatever I could fit into them. I had a dilemma. All of my shoes took up an entire box. Then it hit me. My new life would have to begin with whatever I could fit in these boxes. Whatever I took with me would be what I bring from my past into my future. I had to contemplate carefully on what I felt was irreplaceable. What did I feel was essential? Did I take clothes for interviews and possibly work? Did I take clothes for the Florida summer? What about all the other things I would need? Household things, like forks and towels and pictures and those things I had saved from my kids since pre-school? I had to deconstruct the last twenty years and pack them up in these three boxes.

There were so many things I had attachments to. So many things held emotional sentiment; pictures, gifts from my kids, and from friends and family throughout the years. How would I choose from all of this, what was truly important to me? How was I supposed to sort through the rubble of this crumbled tower called my life? What would I walk away with as my parting gift for participating in this game of life?

M. Rene Harris

CHAPTER NINETEEN

A Recipe for Insanity

"Something powerfully intrinsic happens when the courage to no longer be silent awakens within us and we are compelled to confront our problems rather than cower to them." ~ *Jason Versey*

The garage sale day, for nearly everything we owned, was tomorrow. I had packed up those things that I felt I would need for my immediate future, along with those things that held sentimental value to me. I closed up the boxes, taped them shut, and put the shipping labels on them. Albert was already awake and starting to load items into the trailer. When he wasn't looking, I tucked items that I couldn't pack into the back of the trailer in hopes that someday, I would get them back.

I didn't make any coffee; instead, I stopped at Starbucks on my way to take the boxes to the post office. I kept a pack of cigarettes in my car, and as I drove I opened the pack to have a smoke with my coffee. When I opened the pack a small folded note fell into my lap. Stopped at a stop light, I opened the note and it read "I will kill you." I couldn't decipher the handwriting because it was small - small enough to be put on a tiny piece of paper folded in a pack of cigarettes. The handwriting was neat, neater than any teenager could write, and I had to assume it was Albert. My left brain and my right brain struggled to find the appropriate meaning. Was he going to kill me or were the cigarettes going to kill me?

If Albert was threatening to kill me, then he better do it soon because I was no longer afraid of him and his threats meant nothing to me anymore. I put the note in my glove box, just in case. If anything were to happen to me, the police would find the note and analyze the handwriting and this jerk would rot in prison. If he tried anything, and I survived, I would take the note to the judge and he would be arrested for threatening to murder me. I decided I would hand over the note on Monday morning if I survived the weekend.

The landlord called while I was out running my errands. She found someone who wanted to rent the house and wanted to have them come by in the early evening. The day had progressed quickly as I had spent the majority of it cleaning, organizing and pricing the items that we were selling. The couple arrived that evening and they were very excited about the house. He was a police officer and she was a nurse. They looked around and asked what was staying and what was going. They wanted the refrigerator and the BBQ grill that was fairly new as I had purchased them earlier that year. I told them it could stay, but it was for sale. He paid me for the grill and the fridge, and I placed a "Sold" sign on them. They were nice people and I had the desire to clean the grill and the fridge for them.

As the evening was winding down, I was watching a Disney movie on the TV in the living room with Lily and Steven while waiting for the older two boys, John and Clark, to get home from a play at school. John had just gotten his driver's license and was so excited to be able to drive alone all the way to the high school and back with his brother. The high school was less than five miles away and the play would only last a couple of hours, and since John was in the cast and crew, it would probably take an additional hour for setup and teardown. I didn't get a feeling in my gut, no quickening in my spirit before I heard the horrifying sound of screeching tires and the sound of metal crashing against metal. No internal alarm, but when I heard the crash - I knew. I jumped up from the couch causing Lily to fall to the floor as I ran for the front door. I looked around, then I saw it - right at the turn that leads into the housing area where our home was situated on the corner - my car - my kids.

I ran into the street calling their names with tears streaming down my eyes. My heart was pounding out of my chest. John came running from the car towards me and caught me in his arms. "Mom, we're okay!" I looked at his face and touched his cheek checking for blood then I looked around him towards the mangled cars - I didn't see Clark. I tried to break away from John as he was telling me to calm down, that they were alright. But I didn't see Clark.

I looked towards the house and saw Albert standing there with Lily and Steven - he had no emotion on his face. He didn't ask if anyone was hurt or offer to help. He made no attempt to call the police. Then he said to me, "I hope you kept up your insurance."

I broke away from John and ran to the car. Clark then stepped out of the car and held on to me whispering in my ear "I'm okay, Mom, it's okay." I buried my face into my son's chest and cried, and he held me for a moment before going to the other car to see if the driver or anyone else in the car was hurt.

John had called the police to report the accident, and we began taking pictures of the damage. The driver of the other car was a young pregnant woman who was texting while driving and hit my boys as they were turning onto our street. Clark was telling the police officer in the report that he tried to stop, but the car wouldn't stop - that it seemed like the brakes didn't work. He went on to say that he had a hard time breaking on the way to the school and that's why he figured he better just come straight back home so that I could have them checked.

"Dude, you totaled mom's car!" I would overhear John tell Clark.

Albert had nothing to say - he never asked the kids if they were okay. He never inquired if the other driver was okay. He showed no emotion and that was frightening. I called AAA and they towed the car to the dealership. I would hear the next morning that the car was a total loss. That night I had trouble sleeping and wondered why this man seemed to hate me so much. I cried myself to sleep praying for the protection of my children through all of this madness.

The day of the garage sale I tried my best to get and keep myself under control. I cleaned up what I could muster the energy to clean. Got myself a shower and got dressed and prepared for the people that would come to buy my past. The mother of one of John's friends had prepared some food for us and brought it over. We exchanged information and promised to stay in touch since our boys were such good friends.

I was sitting on the front porch when cars started to arrive. One car pulled up and three black women got out, two older women and one younger, and I could hear one of them say, "That must be her." I could only imagine what they had heard about me. These were some of the friends of Albert's from work. As they approached the house, I said hello and welcomed them, telling them to go right in, that Albert was inside. I stayed sitting on the porch and finished smoking my cigarette before going in and showing them around and make sure nothing was taken without payment.

I went inside and greeted the ladies again, asking if I could show them around, offering them something to drink. The older ladies were very nice and conversed with me - the younger one, late 30s maybe, had no conversation for me whatsoever. I knew in that moment who she was and what she was to Albert. I had excused myself to the bathroom when I heard them speaking amongst themselves.

"I don't know what he's talking about, she's good people."

"She sure is and I'm not about to feed into this mess."

"She's good people," I heard the more aggressive older woman tell Albert.

I went upstairs into my bathroom and looked in the mirror. "I'm good people," I said to myself. I took a deep breath and went back downstairs to finish being a gracious hostess. One of the older women was leaving, I am assuming it was the one who said she wasn't about to feed into this mess. I felt grateful that she saw my heart and hugged her as she left. She wished me luck and blessings.

The younger woman had gone out to the back patio where Albert was sitting and drinking and sat out there with him. More people had started to arrive and leave. Many said they would return with trucks for the larger furniture. The afternoon went by quickly, and we had sold all the larger items, beds, tables, couch, and chairs. Not for a lot, but at least they were going into homes where they would be cared for and put to use. Albert wanted to keep all the money and convinced me he needed it because he would be on the road with the kids and would need to feed them and have enough for gas and emergencies. I agreed for the kids' sake.

It was dark now and Albert was still on the back patio playing music loudly - rap music of all things. The other older woman had left, but the younger woman stayed behind. A few of Alberts other friends stayed for a while, listening to loud music, drinking and getting high. I was embarrassed because this was a nice neighborhood and the association had rules about this type of thing.

As his little going away party ended, everyone had left except the young woman who didn't want to speak to me. I had put the two youngest kids to bed already, and Clark had just come home from a friend's house, but John still wasn't home. He was out with his friends and I had been trying to reach him most of the day. I asked his brother Clark to reach him and tell him to come home. Albert and this younger woman had finally turned off the loud music and come inside, thinking I had gone to bed as well. He asked me why I was still up. "John isn't home and I don't know where he is."

"He's out saying goodbye to his friends, he'll turn up soon."

I went upstairs without turning off any lights or locking any doors, knowing that Albert was right about John, but believing that he was also preparing to take his little girlfriend home. I put Steven into his own bed and crawled into mine with Lily, and as I lay there a strange and icky feeling came over me. I took a deep breath and thought "He's not taking this chick home; he thinks he's going to bang her - right here in my house." I heard myself say out loud, "Oh, hell no!" I got up, got dressed and marched myself downstairs. All the lights were out. Albert and the young woman were in his bedroom. I felt the heat of anger grow inside my stomach. I went to his bedroom and opened the door. He was in bed under the covers without clothes on and she was sitting on the bed still fully clothed. The lights were out and the radio was playing. I took his truck keys from his dresser.

"Come on, Ms. Thing, I'm taking you home right now."

I walked into the hallway thinking that she would be walking quickly behind me. She wasn't.

This bitch was taking her time and I didn't have time for that.

"Ma'am, you have two ways of leaving this house right now. One is to go outside and get in that truck and let me take you home and the other option you don't want. I promise you that."

"I told him to take me home, but he said no." She whispered fearfully.

"Albert, you're an asshole," I said to him. "Come on, I'm not going to hurt you, I'm just taking you to your house or wherever you want to go because you cannot stay here."

"This is not just your house," Albert yelled to me.

"Oh yes, it is you stupid motherfucker, your name is not on the lease or on any bills anywhere and you don't pay for any of it. I do and that makes it mine, you simple piece of shit."

"Let's go before things get real ugly up in here," I said, this time standing in her face.

"Put my keys down." Albert yelled from under the covers.

"Come and get 'em." I snapped back.

He knew better. She followed me out to Albert's truck and got in. I got in and started the truck and pulled out of the housing area onto the main road.

"Which way am I going?" I realized that I had no idea where I was going. I just started driving. She gave me directions to get to her home. She lived over an hour away. Since we had such a long drive ahead of us, I told her everything about him. Everything that he had done over the years, the drugs, the rape, court hearings - everything! I think I was venting and releasing everything that had built up. I told her how he didn't work for years and lived off me until he made me lose my job.

I told her about his porn addiction and that he watched it on the family computer and that he was so uncaring about it that the kids couldn't even do homework without the images popping up on the screen. I told her about the death threat in my pack of cigarettes and the other times I thought he was trying to kill me, but I had no evidence. I told her about the paint in the driveway and in my car. I told her about the kids' car accident and how he just stood there and never bothered to even ask if they were alright or call the police to report it.

She didn't talk much, she just listened. I had an hour of open road at two in the morning, so I just talked. She finally said that the way that Albert had talked about me, she thought I was a white woman. When she saw me sitting on the porch as they pulled up, she thought something must be wrong with me because no black woman was going to let her husband bring another woman up in her house - divorced or not.

"I didn't know anything about you. When Albert said he was going to let some friends come over to pick out some things, I was okay with that," I confessed.

" He told me you knew everything," she replied.

"Nope - I knew he was screwing around, you're not the first. But this is the first time he brought one home." I meant it to be a nasty and cutting remark. Like she was no better than a stray dog that he found.

She was scared. She had every reason to be scared, but I wasn't angry at her. She was a non-issue. I was completely disrespected and so was she. I dropped her off at the house she gave me directions to and now it was time for me to find my way home. I didn't even bother to get her name. I felt kinda bad for that. I prayed all the way home. I prayed for strength. I prayed for the healing of my heart. I prayed for my children. I prayed that John was safe, wherever he was. I prayed for guidance. I prayed for forgiveness for the way I frightened this young woman. She didn't know, she was lied to. She was innocent. How could he do that to her? How could he put her in that kind of situation? But it was Albert, after all, a narcissistic psychopath with no empathy or emotion for anyone except himself.

I offered a prayer of gratitude for the protection that had been given me throughout all of this. Had he been successful in trying to take my life, I wouldn't be here right now, surviving. But I survived. I was protected, I was guided and, in fact, I was blessed.

I found my way back home and parked the truck without causing any damage to it. I had to toss rocks at the boys' window to wake them up to let me in because Albert had locked me out and his set of keys did not have a house key on them. Clark came down and opened the door for me. I thanked him and instructed him to go back to bed. I checked their bedroom, and John was laid sprawled out on his bed asleep. Steven and Lily were still sleeping soundly. I got into bed and went to sleep. I would be leaving in 12 hours.

M. Rene Harris

CHAPTER TWENTY

The Beginning of the End

"The feeling is less like an ending than just another starting point." ~ *Chuck Palahniuk*

I didn't sleep very well, and despite all of my praying, I still felt very angry when I woke up. Not angry for the disrespect Albert had once again shown towards me, but angry at the position he put that woman in by inviting her to my home and then refusing to take her home to coerce her into having sex with him. I wondered why I had married him. Why didn't I run on my wedding day like I wanted to? What would my life be like now if I had? Would I have met the man of my dreams and lived a wonderful life or would I have met someone worse?

What did I ever see in him? I couldn't remember anymore. I couldn't remember what made me fall for him in the first place. I couldn't remember any good times. I can't remember ever having loved him. How did I let it get this far and why did I stay so long? I wondered if I had just left when the boys were little how my life would have turned out. Would we have suffered poverty? Would it have been easier to suffer without him? Was I the best wife that I could have been? Was there anything else I could have done to make it work – to make him love me? Why couldn't he just love me? What is wrong with me? I couldn't find any good reason to justify trying to even be nice to him. It was too late – too much had happened and I no longer knew the man I married. I don't think that I ever really knew him at all.

He told me once that he married me because I told him that I was pregnant. Not sure how that could have been true because we married right after I graduated boot camp and there was no way for me to get pregnant during boot camp. Why did he want to marry me anyway? Maybe he saw me as a meal ticket since he wasn't really ambitious and never really aspired to do or be anything great. He was just there. There breathing and taking up oxygen from good people. There doing nothing. There being nothing but trouble. How would we build a future if I was the only one working towards it? I wanted a future for myself and my children. I wanted them to see the world and all of the wonderful things it had to offer. I wanted them to try different foods. Meet different people and experience different cultures. I wanted them to be rich in experience. I was never going to accomplish that as long as I was with him. His own father told me that years ago.

Now, everything I had worked for was gone. All the money I had was gone. My 401k was depleted, and my marriage is over – I lost my job and now I'm leaving my kids with a man who would rather see me dead than happy. Would a good mother leave her kids behind? What else could I do? I had no job, I could not afford to continue to live in this house since I lost my job and I was tired. My spirit was weary. I was defeated. But at least I'm not dead.

As I lay there asking myself these self-defeating questions, the tears rolled down my cheeks. My plans to have a better life had backfired on me. My thought process was shifting. Better questions were starting to form in my mind. How could I possibly be a good mother if I am showing my kids a relationship that is detrimental?

How is being miserable the best example of how wonderful life could really be?

How was walking on eggshells every single day the makings of a happy family? My fear was gone.

I took a deep breath and wiped my eyes. I needed to end my pity party, put on my big girl panties and get ready to catch a flight to Florida. I went in the bathroom and looked in the mirror. "You are stronger than you know. You are doing the right thing. Things will get better," I repeated to myself before jumping in the shower.

I got dressed and finished packing my suitcases; I would take three large ones and attempt to take two carry-ons and a large purse. Just about everything I owned and called dear had to fit into what I could carry and what I sent in those three large boxes. Whatever I could stash in the trailer for Albert to take unknowingly. It would take a miracle for me to get those things again if he discovered them. But I had to hope. There were so many things that my mother had left to me including the mink coat that Albert had to be ordered by the judge to eventually return to me.

I went downstairs and Albert was already in the kitchen. I wasn't going to say anything, but my mouth seemed to have a mind of its own and my throat felt as if it would burst if I didn't let the words out.

"You owe your friend an apology, Albert. You should have never put her in that situation last night."

"I talked to Clark this morning and asked him if he thought I did anything wrong and he said he didn't think I did anything wrong."

"Well, the first thing you did wrong was asking a 16-year-old if you did anything wrong by bringing your girlfriend into your family's home and then refusing to take her home so that you could have sex with her."

He sat down at the dining room table and put his head down as he listened to my words.

"She seemed like a nice lady and you shouldn't have done that to her. You put her in an awkward position, you put me in an awkward position, even though I know you don't care about that - and you put yourself in the position of some sort of a predator in your kid's eyes. You probably don't care about that either, do you?"

He kept his head down.

"Think about a man who would put our daughter - YOUR daughter in that position. She wants to go home - he's lying in the bed naked trying to get what he wants - she's in another woman's house and he's refusing to take her home. Think about that - marinate on that shit for a minute - now go ask your 16-year-old son again, if you were wrong."

He stayed sitting there with his head down. I didn't care how he felt. I went back upstairs and made sure that I had packed all of my toiletries and checked one last time in all the drawers and cabinets to make sure nothing was left. I would be flying out today, and Albert and the kids would be on the road tomorrow for the long trip to Michigan.

The kids were starting to wake up and we spent time just sitting together, hugging each other and talking about what it would be like when they get to Florida. They wanted to know why they couldn't go with me now. I did my best to explain the cost of the airline tickets, the fact that I would be crashing with their aunt until I found us a home. I assured them that I would not rest until they were back home with me and I promised them that they would have fun spending the summer with their grandparents, aunts, uncles, and cousins in Michigan. I reminded them that there were lakes for fishing and fire pits in the evenings for smores and hotdogs. I forced a smile and a half-hearted laughed, but I think they could sense the disingenuous energy coming from me. I wanted them with me. I wanted it so badly it felt as if my heart was being torn from my chest.

I instructed the boys to bring down my luggage, and I called a cab for the airport. Lily and I sat there hugging and I soothed her cries the best I could while trying not to cry myself. But I couldn't help it. I couldn't stop the tears from streaming down my eyes as I said goodbye to my babies. I did one final check of the house and made sure that all of the keys were in the kitchen drawer as I had promised the landlord they would be. I took the key to the side door, placed it in an envelope and put it on the small island in the middle of the kitchen. I wanted to make sure that everything was in place and that nothing would be forgotten when Albert and the kids left.

I went over the instructions once again with Albert with Clark present. Not that he would be held accountable to his son but just so that I was making myself clear for accountability sake.

"The house needs to be locked up tight when you all leave tomorrow. This key to the side door is to be put in the box outside next to the side door". I held up the envelope that held the key.

"We got this, Mom," Clark assured me, but it wasn't his assurance that I needed.

"The BBQ grill and the fridge stays, it's been sold to the people who will be renting the house," I continued as I looked at Albert for reassurance that he would do the right thing. He looked back at me emotionless. I could not visualize in my mind what was going to happen to this house – to these things – after I was gone.

"Don't worry, Mom," Clark said softly as he gave me a hug. Albert just walked away, saying nothing. I had no faith that he would do the right thing, but I had to trust him. I shouldn't have put the pressure on my son to make his father do the right thing. I knew he didn't have any authority or power.

While the kids were standing there in the kitchen with me holding Lily in my arms, I reminded Albert again to lock the house up and leave this envelope in the box next to the side door for the landlord and the new tenants. He said he would and I asked the boys to make sure that he did. They said they would.

My taxi arrived and honked outside of the front door. I held and kissed my babies' goodbye. Lily didn't want to let me go - her little arms held tightly around my neck as Clark pulled her from me. Albert just stood there looking stupid. The last sight of my children would be them standing in the doorway with tears in their eyes waving goodbye.

My oldest holding my youngest as she cried for me and reached both arms out to be held by me. The taxi driver loaded my bags into the trunk of the cab. I got in the back seat and off we went to the airport. After the kids were out of sight, I sat back in the seat of the cab and took a deep breath. I straightened my shoulders and dried my tears. I had a new focus now. Getting my children home: wherever that was going to be. I had a new mission and I had to make a plan. A well thought out, detailed plan to get my babies because I knew in my gut, that I was going to need one.

Flies in My Coffee

EPILOGUE

Fearless Movement Forward

I wish I could tell you that I lived happily ever after and escaped the mental torment that came from my marriage. But that was not the case, at first. During my first year in Florida, I got my own place and began to replace the things that I had left behind. The battle that ensued from seeking a divorce and finding an amicable solution for custody of the kids lasted for a few more years. Albert and I would eventually divorce and he would remarry and start a new family.

After a year sabbatical, I secured a position at a hotel and focused heavily on my work and securing a new life for me and the kids. Focusing on my career and my children was only the beginning of my transition to finding the inner peace I had been searching for.

Even though I had uprooted everything in our lives and moved across the country, there I was, faced with myself.

I found that I was still holding onto all of the hurt and anger that brought me to this place. I had to ask myself how long I would hold onto this pain turned anger, turned hatred. In order for my true healing to take place and to really empower myself, I would have to learn to let go and forgive. I was confronted with learning what true forgiveness was. But wouldn't forgiving mean that I had to forget? On the contrary. Even though I just wanted to forget everything that happened and show up in my new life a changed person, I couldn't seem to forget all of the injustices I had suffered along the way. Why couldn't I just forget and move on?

I was fortunate enough to be able to remove myself from it physically and now I needed to remove myself from it mentally. Identifying exactly what it was that hurt me meant it was time to assign the blame appropriately and balance the scales.

As I sat still to listen for the answers, I realized that I still had some major work to do on me. I learned that I didn't have to forget. In fact, Forgiveness has nothing to do with forgetting. It has everything to do with remembering. No wound can transcend into forgiveness with the remembrance of it. That's how we learn not to touch hot stoves a second time. That is how we learn not to repeat detrimental or harmful patterns. Remembering the past from a victim mentality is what keeps us from being able to forgive. We give any hurtful memory the energy conducive to un-forgiveness when we come at it like that. Remembering the past while putting those events in a perspective outside of my injured self, allowed me to begin to move beyond it. Unforgiveness, hurt and unresolved anger can be paralyzing and keep us in a state of not being able to move on with our lives. I begin to develop a need to forgive as a way of healing the rupture. I began closing the gap of the injury that took place by acceptance. By accepting that there was a violation of trust, naming those violations and releasing with them one by one, I slowly released myself from being held hostage to past events. Those memories no longer held the weight they once did. They no longer held the level of pain that kept them fresh in my mind.

My trust was betrayed. I trusted that someone I loved would never hurt me. We all go into relationships with that unspoken agreement. My trust was shattered and it broke me emotionally. I had to come to terms with my part as well. I allowed bad behavior by not firmly setting boundaries and sticking to what I would and would not tolerate early on in the relationship. I had to accept and forgive myself for breaking trust with my own internal guidance system.

Setting myself free from this torment meant setting him free. I had to release him from owing me anything to amend the wrong he had done. As long as I felt he owed me something, I kept him indebted to me and I kept myself bankrupt. Without removing myself from this mental prison, I knew I would forever be trapped in this perpetual cycle of victimhood. I alone held the power to free myself. I absolved his debt to me. The moment that I made that choice, I also forgave myself. It was like a thousand pounds had been lifted from me.

Without forgiveness, I would not be able to emerge into my fierce new self. Living fearlessly, means that my life didn't have to revolve around my past.

I am not a victim because I choose not to be. We can go from victim to rescuer, and then martyr in a vicious cycle that never seems to end in the name of sacrificing ourselves for the greater good of everyone else but ourselves. I had assumed the role long before I got married. I subconsciously brought it into my marriage, my job and every other situation in my life until I learned that enough was enough and a little was too much. We all deserve peace and happiness in this lifetime. We have survived the worst so that we can be our best. For that, I am grateful.

It is with gratitude that I greet each day. Grateful for guidance and peace within and the ability to recognize that as much as my suffering was an inside job, so was my peace.

M. Rene Harris

ABOUT THE AUTHOR

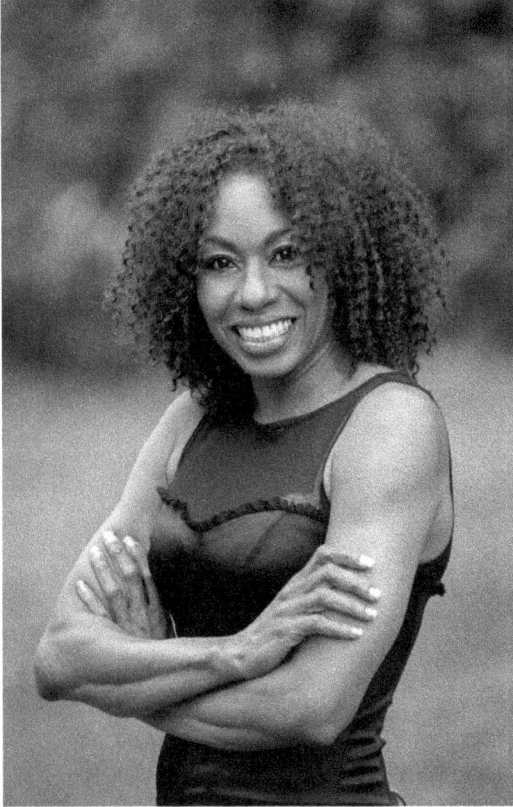

M. Rene Harris is a speaker and international traveler who has worked in the Spa and Wellness field of Hospitality for nearly two decades. She is a Certified Naturopathic Nutritionist and holds a BA in Business Management. As a former U.S. Marine and mother of four she believes that while meditation practice, physical fitness and healthy eating are important; mental stress is the number one cause of disease, premature aging and death. This belief is what ignited this spa maven's passion for peace. M. Rene currently resides with her family and their dog, Fat Kitty, in Tampa Bay, Florida.

M. Rene Harris

RICHTER
PUBLISHING

www.ingramcontent.com/pod-product-compliance
Lightning Source LLC
Chambersburg PA
CBHW052126270326
41930CB00012B/2778